PRAISE FOR

# *A Teen's Guide to Gut Health*

"Rachel Meltzer Warren handles this delicate topic with honesty and humor, delivering an empowering plan of action that's heavy on evidence-based, practical solutions to redirect readers from the rabbit hole of unvetted, fad-driven online advice."

—TAMARA DUKER FREUMAN, MS, RD, CDN, clinical dietitian, contributor, *U.S. News & World Report*

"This unique book will help you manage your IBS in a school setting, including specific strategies for managing your social life, access to the bathroom, cafeteria, dorm living and going out to eat with your friends. I love the laugh-out-loud scripts for talking to parents about IBS!"

—PATSY CATSOS, MS, RDN, LD, author of *The IBS Elimination Diet and Cookbook*

"What a terrific resource! This comprehensive guide covers all the bases. Complete with delicious recipes and sample meal plans, this is the go-to GI guide for all teens and young adults."

—FAYE BERGER MITCHELL, RDN, LDN, editor-in-chief, *foodieoncampus.com*

"For any teen who is struggling to understand what's going on in their gut, this book is a must read!"

—NANCY SIDNAM, MS, RDN, creator of The Wellie Project

"*A Teen's Guide to Gut Health* will prove to be a life-changing resource for adolescents who are looking to get their young lives back to normal."

—DR. BARBARA BOLEN, coauthor of *The Everything Guide to the Low-FODMAP Diet*

ALSO BY RACHEL MELTZER WARREN

*The Smart Girl's Guide to Going Vegetarian*

# A Teen's Guide to GUT HEALTH

# A Teen's Guide to GUT HEALTH

## The LOW-FODMAP Way
### TO TAME IBS, CROHN'S, COLITIS, and OTHER DIGESTIVE DISORDERS

### RACHEL MELTZER WARREN, MS, RDN

THE EXPERIMENT

NEW YORK

The Experiment, LLC
220 East 23rd Street, Suite 301
New York, NY 10010-4674
www.theexperimentpublishing.com

The Experiment's books are available at special discounts when purchased in bulk for premiums and sales promotions as well as for fund-raising or educational use. For details, contact us at info@theexperimentpublishing.com.

Library of Congress Cataloging-in-Publication

Names: Warren, Rachel Meltzer, author.
Title: A teen's guide to gut health : the low-FODMAP way to tame IBS,
    Crohn's, colitis, and other digestive disorders / Rachel Meltzer Warren,
    MS, RDN.
Description: New York : The Experiment, [2017]
Identifiers: LCCN 2016020920 (print) | LCCN 2016026265 (ebook) | ISBN
    9781615193547 (pbk) | ISBN 9781615193554 (ebook)
Subjects: LCSH: Gastrointestinal system--Diseases--Popular works. |
    Gastrointestinal system--Diseases--Diet therapy. | Teenagers--Health and
    hygiene--Popular works.
Classification: LCC RC806 .W37 2017 (print) | LCC RC806 (ebook) | DDC
    641.5/631--dc23
LC record available at https://lccn.loc.gov/2016020920

ISBN 978-1-61519-354-7
Ebook ISBN 978-1-61519-355-4

Cover and text design by Becky Terhune
Author photograph by Daniel Meltzer

Manufactured in the United States of America
Distributed by Workman Publishing Company, Inc.
Distributed simultaneously in Canada by Thomas Allen & Son Ltd.

First printing January 2017
10 9 8 7 6 5 4 3 2 1

*To my parents, who gave me my guts*

# CONTENTS

# FOREWORD

Gastrointestinal (GI) problems are remarkably common, disruptive, and embarrassing. Let's face it: It can be pretty awkward to talk about your own or hear about other's problems with stomach gurgling, farting, or pooping. Perhaps the most common and best-known GI problem is irritable bowel syndrome or IBS—a condition characterized by symptoms such as abdominal pain, bloating, and altered bowel habits (diarrhea and/or constipation). Doctors will tell you that the good news is that IBS won't kill you. Patients will tell you that the bad news is that IBS won't kill you. . . .

Because IBS is considered a nonlethal "lifestyle condition," it often isn't taken seriously by doctors, teachers, coaches, friends, or even family. But fun everyday activities for most teens—like participating in or attending sporting events, dating, or eating out at a restaurant—can become sources of fear, frustration, anxiety, and isolation for those with IBS.

By the way, the common denominator for many social activities is *food*. Consider how the role of food in everyday life has changed over the roughly two-hundred-thousand-year existence of humankind. For most of history, food has predominantly been viewed as a source of sustenance and nutrition. In the past, if someone wanted food to eat, they had to grow or hunt it (even in less developed parts of the world today, food is not always easily available). If someone got a headache or a cut, they couldn't go to the corner drugstore to pick up some acetaminophen or antibiotic ointment. Rather, they counted upon the healing properties of plant and animal products. Now fast-forward to modern times in developed areas. Food can sometimes be less about sustenance and nutrition and more about pleasure and entertainment. So many things that we do involve food as a major part of the overall experience, and in some ways, food can be readily available with little effort. Think about how you planned your days the last time you went on vacation with your family—I bet it was around mealtimes! For Americans, it isn't unusual to talk about where you're going to eat dinner while you're eating lunch. Whether you view that as comical or just plain sad, there can be no denying that we have strayed quite far from the words of the ancient philosopher and physician Hippocrates, who said, "Let food be your medicine and medicine be your food."

Increasingly, health care providers are waking up to the fact that the majority of GI problems are related to what we eat. For example, it has long been known that two thirds of IBS patients link eating a meal with their GI symptoms. Yet despite this fact, meaningful research to identify scientifically proven dietary treatments for conditions like IBS has been hard to find. This lack of scientific evidence, along with patients' urgent need for relief, has created an environment that is ripe for unfounded and, in some cases, even dangerous diet treatments. It is precisely for that reason that *A Teen's Guide to Gut Health* is so important. Over the past eight years or so, there has been an explosion of scientific research dedicated to unraveling the role of diet in causing and treating GI symptoms. There is now credible evidence that supports the benefits of the low-FODMAP diet in patients with IBS. This book does a great job of weaving the available scientific evidence, common sense, and the invaluable experience of author Rachel Meltzer Warren to create an informative, medically responsible, and entertaining journey to Dietary Nirvana for teens with GI conditions. By using this book, teens with IBS, inflammatory bowel disease (IBD), or other GI disorders can gain the knowledge and tools necessary to enjoy the parts of life involving food that they have been missing.

**WILLIAM D. CHEY**
MD, AGAF, FACG, FACP, RFF

Timothy T. Nostrant Collegiate Professor of
  Gastroenterology and Nutrition Sciences
Director, Digestive Disorders Nutrition and
  Lifestyle Program
Director, GI Physiology Laboratory
Division of Gastroenterology
University of Michigan Health System
Ann Arbor, Michigan

# INTRODUCTION

I t can be hard enough to feel comfortable in your own skin as a teenager in this Instagram-perfect, status-updated world we're living in. And if you have chronic digestive problems or have been diagnosed with a gut disorder like irritable bowel syndrome (IBS), Crohn's disease, ulcerative colitis, or another condition that forces you to become better than Google Maps when it comes to finding a toilet (and fast!), that challenge is even greater.

Maybe you've lost your focus during an important exam because the teacher wouldn't let you get out to the bathroom. Or declined an invitation for a sleepover or school trip because you're worried your stomach will make embarrassing noises when you least expect it. Perhaps you've wandered the cafeteria, wondering which of the limited food options won't make your symptoms act up, or wished there were something else you could do to find relief but don't know where to turn. And while loads of adults have the same digestive problems, they also typically have more control when it comes to using the restroom, choosing the right foods, and getting help.

That's exactly why I wanted to write this book. Roughly 14 percent of high school students in the United States have the symptoms of IBS; even more young people are affected when you consider those with diagnoses of the inflammatory bowel diseases (Crohn's disease and ulcerative colitis), and other less common issues. If you're one of those millions of young people affected, you may not know where to turn.

My first goal with this book is to help you figure out what's going on with your insides—giving you an easy-to-understand primer on gut health so you have the vocabulary you need to discuss digestion without reverting to words you learned in preschool, and so you know what to expect from doctors' visits and any medical testing you might need. I made sure it's packed with real-life advice and tips from teens who've been there, so you know you're not alone and so you can learn from their experiences.

The second goal is to spread the word about the low-FODMAP plan, an amazing, effective diet that helps diminish or eliminate symptoms in as many as 86 percent of people with IBS—as well as those with Crohn's disease, ulcerative colitis, and celiac disease—and make it not a total snooze fest for young people to read about. As a registered dietitian nutritionist (RDN), I've seen clients of all ages struggle with digestive troubles, with few remedies that work. When I started recommending the low-FODMAP plan, I was simply blown away. The name is funny (I'll explain it later), but for the majority of people with IBS and plenty of folks with other digestive disorders, it works. Follow this plan and you'll up your chances of living a normal, healthy life. I've broken it down in a way that you can easily implement—at home, at school, and on the go.

I hope you enjoy the stories, the information, and the recipes. But most of all, I hope you feel well.

From the bottom of my gut,
Rachel

## What Is a Registered Dietitian Nutritionist?

A registered dietitian nutritionist (RDN), also sometimes known as a registered dietitian (RD), is a health professional who specializes in using food and nutrition to promote wellness. People with the letters *RDN* after their names have, at a minimum, a bachelor's degree or the equivalent courses in nutrition and dietetics, have completed a roughly yearlong supervised practice or internship program to learn from registered dietitian nutritionists in hospitals and other settings, have passed a national certifying exam (sort of like the bar exams lawyers take, but with a whole lot of chemistry instead of legal stuff), and constantly earn continuing education credits to keep up on the latest in the field. It's true: We're nerds. But we're nerds who love good food and helping people feel their best.

## CHAPTER 1

# Getting to Know Your Gut

**B**efore you can understand what might be wrong with your digestion and how to fix it, you need to understand what happens when things are working well: how food makes the epic journey from your plate to the parts of your body that use it, and how you get rid of the foodstuffs you don't need along the way.

The GI or gastrointestinal tract begins with your mouth and ends with your rectum. Whether you're a Kourtney or Khloé height-wise, your GI tract clocks in at up to thirty feet long as you approach adult size—when it's spread out from one end to the other, that is. This winding tube is lined with smooth muscle that helps any food you eat travel from your mouth to your stomach and intestines, and out the other side. We'll get into the specifics of the role that each part plays soon—but for now, think about it as one long tube.

The craziest thing you may ever learn about your digestive tract: It's technically located outside of your body. Sure, you've never glanced down in the middle of history class and seen it looking up at you. But any part of your body that has contact with the world around you is considered ever so technically by medical professionals to be outside the body. Your bones, for instance, protected by skin, muscle, and more, are inside. Your brain, protected by your skull and skin, is inside. Your lips mostly keep your mouth covered . . .

but open that doorway to let some food or drink in and *bam*—your digestive tract is up close and personal with the outside world. And technically, anything that passes through your digestive tract remains outside of your body until it's broken down and absorbed by the small intestine into the bloodstream (stay tuned for details on how that works).

## THE JOURNEY TO POOP

So how does food make the epic journey from your mouth through this winding tube called the digestive tract, sending important nutrients out to your body and anything that's left over out the other end? When I ask my clients what the first step of the digestion process is, they usually tell me that it's when you swallow food or when it reaches your stomach. Most are surprised to hear that digestion begins before you've eaten a single thing.

### The First Step

Have you ever felt your mouth water when you're waiting for a hot slice of pizza to come out of the oven? This process—technically called *salivation*— is part of your body readying itself for incoming food. (This is also why you might feel the urge to tackle your brother when he pops the last tater tot—which

you were totally just about to eat—into his mouth.)

When you finally do take that first bite of food, the saliva you've already produced is at the ready to help soften what you've eaten so your teeth can break it down into an easy-to-swallow mush. In addition to turning food into a mass that can effortlessly slide down your throat, saliva contains digestive enzymes that work chemically to start turning nutrients into smaller components. One enzyme, called *salivary amylase,* chemically helps break down long chains of carbohydrates. If you put a piece of a carbohydrate-rich food like bread in your mouth and let it sit there, you can actually taste it becoming sweeter as the salivary amylase breaks the carbohydrate down into simple starches, the smaller building blocks that make up carbohydrates. While that happens, another enzyme, called *salivary lipase,* kicks off the process of digesting fats.

Next, you chew, turning your meal from, well, food, into what's called a *bolus*—a word that's Greek and Latin for "lump," and in the case of digestion, refers specifically to a ball of food. Chewing is probably not something you've thought much about since you were an infant learning how to eat solid

## Open, Shut Them

Everything in your body is connected, and your mouth, airway, and nose are no exception. Whether or not you've noticed it, every time you eat something, your nose and throat essentially close their doors so that food stays in your mouth while you chew and break it down. If you've ever had food "go down the wrong pipe" or had a cruel friend make you laugh as you took a swig of lemonade, you know how important it is for everything to cooperate so you don't breathe in (*aspirate*) food, or experience the pleasure of OJ shooting out of your nose. Ew.

food and your parents were standing over you making exaggerated chompy faces to remind you not to swallow your banana whole. But the simple, mindless act of chewing your food deserves some attention even at your advanced age—and here's why: Chewing does more than just ensure you don't choke (though that is, admittedly, pretty important). When you chew, you increase the surface area of your food so that the enzymes produced by your saliva can reach more of what you've eaten and be more effective in breaking it down into smaller pieces. Chewing also signals your stomach to prepare for the food's arrival by releasing acid that will help with digestion. What's more, research shows that chewing for longer can help you feel more satisfied when you eat, and can even help your body absorb more nutrients from food.

As soon as you're ready to swallow, your tongue propels the bolus of food back into your esophagus. The first door (called the *upper esophageal sphincter*, or UES) opens, welcoming the bolus into your esophagus, where a wave known as *peristalsis* carries it downward (with the help of gravity) and through a second door, called the *lower esophageal sphincter* (or LES). The LES separates your esophagus from your stomach.

## The Stomach Scene

Next, the bolus of food finally arrives at the stomach, which can hold as much as four cups (about a liter) of chewed food or liquid, expanding as you eat or drink to accommodate whatever you've taken in. The top part of your stomach serves as a waiting room, where the bolus rests as the lower stomach (called the *antrum*)

# How Many Times Should I Chew?

There's no official number for how many times you should chew to adequately break down food (even though rumors about this seem to circulate the Internet all the time). But chances are, if you live in the same on-the-run, hold-on-while-I-just-send-this-one-Snap world I do, you're eating in a hurry—and not chewing nearly enough. In an effort toward getting the most out of your food, try this exercise:

1. Sit down for a meal or snack with as few distractions as possible. No friends or family to chat with, no apps, no TV. Try to be home so that you can even limit background noise like music or chatter.

2. Take a bite of your food. Chew it thirty times. Notice when you first have the urge to swallow, and whether or not it's difficult to chew so much. Do you have to remind yourself not to swallow?

3. Notice how the food in your mouth has changed. What is the texture like now? What about the flavor?

4. Do the same for the next three mouthfuls. Is chewing thirty times uncomfortable? Why or why not?

5. On the next bite, chew until you feel you've chewed thoroughly—you don't need to reach thirty. What number seems like enough for this particular food?

6. Resume eating normally, with an increased attention to adequate chewing. Revisit this exercise often, preferably at the start of each meal, so that you can reset the speed at which you eat and begin to make chewing thoroughly second nature.

begins to contract and mix the food with enzymes and acids. Hydrochloric acid creates conditions that are at just the right pH (or acidity level) for the digestion of protein as well as the killing off of bacteria, while the enzyme pepsin starts the process of breaking the protein down. The enzyme lipase continues to break down fats. As that happens, the lining of the stomach produces mucus, which will protect it from being harmed by all of that damaging acidity.

Once the bolus has been pummeled by the hydrochloric acid and pepsin, it's now considered *chyme*—a liquefied mass of partially digested food, water, and more. Peristaltic waves continue to move the chyme downward toward the pyloric sphincter (also known as the *pyloric valve*), a ring of muscle that controls the flow of chyme from the lower stomach into the upper small intestine, called the *duodenum*. (It also prevents chyme from bouncing back up into the stomach.) You can think of the pyloric sphincter like the security at the entrance to the Apple Store the day a new iPhone comes out. If the duodenum is at capacity, it's not letting any more food in. As food enters the duodenum, a little opening called the *sphincter of Oddi* funnels in digestive juices from the pancreas and bile from the gallbladder (the latter is produced in the liver). Bile emulsifies fat into smaller pieces, making it available for digestion and absorption, while the enzymes use chemicals to further break down protein, fat, and carbohydrates.

## Beyond the Breakdown

Up until this point, digestion has consisted of taking apart the nutrients in food and turning them into smaller and smaller pieces. We've now reached the stage of digestion in which things begin to get exciting. *Exciting?* you're asking? Yes, exciting! Because, full disclosure, the small intestine is my absolute favorite

digestive organ. It is. (Doesn't everyone have one? No? Oh. Right. Well, I'm going to own this anyway.) The reason I love the small intestine? At its beginning, the process of breaking down food into smaller components is continuing, but by its end, you're actually absorbing nutrients—real, live nutrients!—into your bloodstream, where they are then delivered to the various parts of your body to do the important things that nutrients do, like give you energy, repair your cells, make your bones strong, and so, so much more. The small intestine, in fact, is where most nutrients are absorbed into the bloodstream so that they can move on to do their jobs throughout your body. How cool is that?!

Where was I? Oh yes. So after the chyme passes through the duodenum, peristalsis continues, which helps it stay on its journey. The walls of the small intestine start out as smooth as a bedsheet, but farther along they develop folds called *villi* and *microvilli*, which make them resemble your grandparents' 1970s-era shag carpet that's sorely in need of a makeover. These microscopic hairlike projections increase the surface area of the intestinal lining, which allows for more and better absorption of nutrients. Villi and microvilli line the walls of the remaining two sections of

# Turn Digestion on Its Head

Beginning in your esophagus when you first swallow food, a system of muscular contractions called *peristalsis* works like waves to squeeze the bolus along, moving it through the different parts of your digestive tract. Peristalsis works so well that if you're upside-down doing an handstand and a friend decides to feed you a smoothie through a straw, the drink would still move down your esophagus, through the lower esophageal sphincter, into your stomach, and beyond—and you'd actually feel the GI tract gently contracting to push it along. And then you'd tell your friend to take a hike, because, really, who does that?! But anyway, it's a cool science experiment that will help you never forget what peristalsis is. (Fun fact: We did this exercise in my ninth-grade biology class, and apparently it was a life-altering nerd moment for me, because here I am telling you about it today. And I, too, thought I would never use the things I learned in school!)

the small intestine, the jejunum and ileum. The walls of these parts of the intestine absorb fats and other nutrients; then blood vessels transport those nutrients through the portal vein to the liver. By the time your food reaches the end of the small intestine, most of its nutrients, as well as all but about one liter of fluid, have been absorbed. Another sphincter, called the *ileocecal valve,* separates the small intestine from the large intestine and also keeps chyme from splashing back into the ileum.

The large intestine is also known as the *colon* or the *large bowel*. In healthy people, the chyme is mostly liquid when it enters the large intestine, and mostly solid when it exits the large intestine. So can you guess what the role of the large intestine is? You got it—removing all of that fluid through absorption, which occurs as what's left over from the small intestine makes its journey through the various parts of the colon (from the cecum to the ascending colon to the transverse colon to the descending colon to the sigmoid colon and into the rectum). The large intestine also contains bacteria that, in addition to producing nutrients like vitamin K—the blood-clotting vitamin—further digest any remaining bits of carbohydrate and protein. The balance of bacteria throughout the digestive tract (known as the *gut microbiome*), and in the large intestine in particular, may hold the key to understanding and managing your symptoms; we'll talk about this in great detail throughout the book. Stick with me, friends—before long, you, too, will have your very own fan-favorite digestive organ and tell tales of peristalses past.

## So Long, Number 2

The rectum and anus are where food ends its journey through the digestive tract. The rectum is typically empty, since your sigmoid colon holds on to poop until it's ready to come out. Once the area above the sigmoid colon becomes full, you feel the urge to go—and under the best of healthy circumstances, you can control that urge until you've reached a bathroom. When you're ready, the rectum pushes out the poop through the anus, the opening through which waste exits your body, controlled by a ring of muscle called the anal sphincter.

## DIGESTION: THE MOVIE

Processing and using food depends on much more than the parts of the body that are at the center of the action, however. Digestion is somewhat like the process of making a film. Have you ever watched the credits roll after a big blockbuster? There are thousands of people involved, many with jobs you never knew existed. Digestion, like making a movie, is an uber-collaborative effort that goes way beyond the mouth, stomach, and small and large intestines, which as you now know all play starring roles. The liver, pancreas, and gallbladder are supporting actors, supplying important enzymes and other compounds that help break down food. And behind the scenes, the nervous system is the producer/director, calling the shots and getting everyone to do his job—like stimulating production coordinators saliva and peristalsis, nudging the cleaning team to tidy up with the migrating motor complex (see "Why Grazing Isn't Great" on p. 10). The whole time, bacteria work as the crew to keep things humming along; and like any group working together, some members do the heavy lifting while others kind of get in the way, which you'll learn more about later because it's at the crux of the low-FODMAP plan. Finally, the circulatory system gets those nutrients out to the parts of the body that will use them, much like the film distributor who puts the ready-to-watch movie in theaters for people to go and enjoy.

No doubt, digestion is a major motion picture that involves many players. This is why gut disorders are incredibly common; so many different parts need to align just right for healthy digestion to occur. Now that you have a good understanding of how this happens, we can take a look at what might be up with your body and prepare you for how a doctor might investigate.

FACTS

## Why Grazing Isn't Great

If you're more of a "nosh all day" person than a "three square meals" one, your eating schedule may be contributing to your gut problems. When you haven't eaten in one and half to two hours, a wave of electrical activity called a migrating motor complex (MMC) sweeps through your digestive tract. This action cleans up any leftovers that are still in your gut. It may also make your stomach growl—a rumbling tummy doesn't always mean that you're hungry! If you're constantly snacking, you'll never give your body a chance to activate the MMC, potentially leaving fuel for not-so-good bacteria to grow and thrive on. Stress can also affect the MMC. To ensure regular MMC clean sweeps, work on keeping tension to a minimum (see Chapter 8) and waiting three to five hours between snacks and meals.

# CHAPTER 2

# Getting Diagnosed

**E**verybody's experienced stomach upset at some point. But there's a big difference between having a stomach virus and what you're likely going through if you've picked up this book.

If you've already been diagnosed with a gut disorder, great! Well, not so great . . . that stinks. But I'm glad you know what's causing your discomfort. Knowledge is power—really. So if you've already been diagnosed, you might want to skip ahead to Chapter 3, though it probably wouldn't hurt to read through this chapter at some point, to get some insight into what clues helped your doctor draw his or her conclusion.

## WHEN TO SEE THE DOCTOR

If you haven't been diagnosed, how do you know when it's time to go to the doctor? First things first, you should put this book down and go straight to the emergency room if:

- The pain is so severe you need to curl into a ball or can't sit still.
- You have pain accompanied by persistent nausea, bloody stools, vomiting, yellowed skin, tenderness, and/or swelling in the belly area.
- You are vomiting or pooping blood (especially if it's maroon or tarry black).
- You are unable to pass stool, especially if you are vomiting.
- You have chest, neck, or shoulder pain.
- You have pain in or between your shoulder blades with nausea.

- Your belly is tender or rigid and hard to the touch.
- You've had an injury to your abdominal area.
- You're having a hard time breathing.

If you're not already in the midst of a medical emergency, I strongly recommend making an appointment to see your doctor if you have one or more of these symptoms:

- You have abdominal pain that lasts more than a few days.
- You have loose stools for more than five days.
- You regularly have to run to the bathroom and are worried you might not make it in time.
- You have diarrhea accompanied by signs of dehydration—thirst, dark-colored urine, infrequent urination, dry skin, fatigue, light-headedness, or dizziness.
- You're experiencing constipation or diarrhea along with stomach pain for more than two days.
- You're losing weight without trying.
- You're having severe or persistent gas.
- You're feeling uncomfortably bloated for more than a few days.

- You have any gastrointestinal symptom that is getting in the way of your quality of life.

If you're reading this book, I'm guessing that at minimum you said yes to the last statement. And if that's you, there are two reasons I'm going to urge you to see a doctor. First is to rule out anything serious. Now, I'm not going to get all panicky and say that if you've been having stomach issues it's probably something grave. Chances are, it's not. Digestive problems, it seems, can cause a lot of pain and aggravation without being life threatening—and that's the case for countless people. You know how to Google, so I'm not going to waste trees (or screen space—thanks, e-readers!) in this book outlining the scary conditions you *might* have. The odds are extremely low that you are suffering from something life-threateningly terrible. However, it is important to see a doctor to rule out that very small possibility; you also want to make sure your symptoms aren't being caused by a serious-but-manageable condition like celiac disease, which requires a very specific diet, or something that might need close monitoring, medication, or both.

## SURVIVING AT SCHOOL

"I always dread going to school because of my IBS. Sometimes I text my dad to pick me up."

"I tell myself that this phase will pass, and that I can't let IBS take control of my life."

"I suggest online school while you figure everything out."

"Make sure you talk to your friends and teachers to catch up on any work you may have to miss."

The second reason I want you to see a doctor is something to keep in mind as you embark on this voyage of identifying and improving the causes of your gut symptoms. Three important words: You deserve it. You are entitled to good health. You are worthy of feeling great every day. Your stomach should not be getting in the way of having a happy life. If it is, you need to take action. This book is one piece of a puzzle. I will do everything I can to help you. But nothing written by a person you've never met can match the personal interaction you'll get from meeting with a medical professional. Now, I can't promise you that seeing a physician will end in your getting a

diagnosis and effective treatment. But regardless, it's an important step on your road to wellness and shouldn't be dismissed. You deserve it.

# KEEPING TRACK OF SYMPTOMS

Now, if you looked at the list on p. 12 and thought to yourself, "I don't know! I just know my stomach is *not right*!" you, too, should see a doctor, but you may need to do a little investigative work before you make that appointment. Even if stomach troubles have been taking over your life, it can be hard to remember the details of what's been happening from day to day. That's why it's important that

## OPENING UP

"Don't be afraid to be honest with those who are able to help you."

"I talk to my therapist, because she actually tries to understand me."

"My mom is a registered dietitian; she's good at helping me."

"I tell my friends about my stomach issues so I can get it off my chest. Some of them understand."

"I feel like I can be open with my gastroenterologist."

"My parents are supportive, especially my dad, because he has IBS as well."

you keep a symptom journal, starting as soon as you realize something's off. Or today. Today would be a good day to start, too. The sooner the better, so that when you're face to face with a medical professional, you'll have the context and history you need. You can dedicate a Google Doc to tracking symptoms, keep an email thread to yourself in your "Drafts" folder, or do it the old-fashioned pen-and-paper way. You might also try a more modern—and maybe powerful option—a symptom-tracking app. A free one called My GI Health focuses on concerns about gut health and may even be more complete and useful than a medical history taken by your doctor, according to a study published in the *American Journal of Gastroenterology*

(share it with her, of course, to help improve your communication).

Keeping track of your symptoms is easy once you have your system in place. Write or type the date. If you wake up feeling fine, eat a bowl of Coco Yum-Yum Flakes cereal, and promptly find yourself running to the bathroom with pink-and-purple polka-dotted diarrhea, write that down. Or make a note if you feel bloated and uncomfortable in the middle of a science test. Or if you haven't pooped in five days and you're feeling twisted and heavy. Any type of digestive discomfort is worth writing down. For any symptoms you're recording, rate them on a scale of 1 to 10 (1 being the mildest, 10 the worst). Try to be as descriptive as possible (for example, "sharp pain on right side") and include any other details that might be relevant, such as what you ate or drank, if you're feeling stressed, or (girls) if you're having your period.

## MAKING THE APPOINTMENT

Now, maybe you're the kind of person who tells your parents *everything*. I will always remember one time when I was in college having dinner at a restaurant with a friend's family; her high school–age brother got up to use the restroom and came back to the table announcing that he'd just made a huge poop (pretty sure his language was more colorful), and boy did he feel great now. I turned beet red, but my friend and her parents didn't blink. In fact, they all started talking about how recently they'd pooped, or whether they'd need to later on. The color of my face probably gave it away that this was not dinnertime conversation at my house. OK, so this wasn't *anytime* conversation in my family! Point being: Everyone has a different comfort level with this sort of thing.

Maybe you're used to relatives like my friend's and chatting about your adventures in the loo doesn't faze you one bit. Or maybe your family is like mine and some things are a bit more private. Either way, you need to be able to discuss the fact that you're having some issues with your parents. It can be embarrassing to talk about bathroom issues with anyone. But first remember that nobody loves you more or cares more about your well-being than those people who created you and/or who have raised you. They changed your diapers, so it's no surprise to them that you poop, even if they don't feel the need to talk about it much (thank you, Mom and Dad!).

That said, you don't need to give them the gory details in order to get some help seeing your doctor, which is the goal here. Here are two sample conversations you might have—one with a nervous parent and another with an overly laid-back one—that will help you get your point across while still maintaining some sense of privacy.

### Nervous Parent Script

You: Hey, Mom, can we talk about something?

Mom: Sure!

You: I'd like to make an appointment to see the doctor.

Mom: Why? Is something wrong? Oh my goodness, WHAT'S WRONG?

# What to Say When You're Uncomfortable

It's great if you can use real, adult words when it comes to talking about your body. But if that's hard, it shouldn't get in the way of your getting the help you need. Here are some ways to "talk around" the symptoms with your parents so they will help you get to the doctor.

**DIARRHEA:** "I have to go to the bathroom a lot." "When I go to the bathroom, it's watery."

**URGENCY:** "I'm afraid I won't make it to the bathroom in time."

**BLOODY STOOL:** "I saw blood in the toilet."

**CONSTIPATION:** "I'm having trouble going to the bathroom." "I hardly ever go number two."

**BLOATING:** "My stomach feels puffed up."

**GAS:** "I have a lot of air in my belly."

**You:** Nothing! It's nothing! OK, it's not nothing. But please don't freak out, Mom. I've just been having some issues with my stomach.

**Mom:** Your stomach? Is it ulcers? CANCER? Do you have diarrhea, sweetie? You'd tell me if you had diarrhea, right? Is it bloody? Mucusy? Mucusy and bloody diarrhea?!

**You:** Mom! Calm down. It's just . . . I have to go to the bathroom a lot, and I looked around on the Internet and I think my symptoms sound a little bit like IBS. I'd rather talk about it more with my doctor.

**Mom:** IBS. Oh. Your grandma has that, you know.

**You:** Really? I didn't know that.

**Mom:** But tell me more! How much diarrhea do you have? Are you in pain? Is this why you stayed home from school the other day? Why didn't you tell me sooner?!

**You:** Mom, I will be OK. It is why I stayed home; at first I just thought I ate

## TALKING TO PARENTS

"My parents give me a lot of emotional support, especially when I'm feeling down and just want to stay in my bed."

"I can't talk about it with my dad, that makes me feel uncomfortable."

"I talk to my mom. She has celiac disease, too, so she can give me advice. I also feel comfortable telling her when my stomach hurts."

"I am very shy to talk to anyone about this."

"I talk to my mom or sister because they have the same disease."

something bad, and then I thought I was nervous because of midterms. But it's not getting better. That's why I think the most important thing is that I talk to the doctor to find out what it is for sure and see if there are any tests I should get.

**Mom:** That's probably true. OK. I'm glad we could talk so openly and easily!

**You:** [suppressing eye roll] Thanks, Mom.

## Laid-Back Parent Script

**You:** Hey, Dad, do you have a sec?

**Dad:** Sure.

**You:** I'd like to make an appointment to see the doctor.

**Dad:** Why? Didn't you just go for a checkup a few months back?

**You:** Well, yes. But for the past month or so, my stomach's been bothering me.

**Dad:** Oh, you probably just ate something bad.

**You:** Maybe. But I think that would have passed by now, and I've been feeling not so great for at least four weeks.

**Dad:** All right. Well, you're not throwing up, so it's probably nothing. Let me know if it gets any worse, and we can go to the doctor if the pain acts up.

**You:** Well, it's not exactly painful—more like a constant discomfort. Every day.

Even at school. I'm not in severe pain, but I'm feeling off. I have to go to the bathroom a lot more than normal, and I'm afraid it's getting in the way of classes and soccer practice. I'd really like to talk to the doctor to see if there is anything I can do to make it better. I don't want to jeopardize my grades and performance on the field.

**Dad:** I see. I didn't realize it was getting in the way of your life so much. I'll make an appointment right now.

*Another important note:* There are loads of doctors around who would love to help you. If you don't like or feel comfortable around your current doctor, ask your parents if you can try a new one. The medical professionals in your life should always listen to you and be supportive and easy to talk to. If your current MD doesn't fit the bill, keep shopping.

## WHAT TO EXPECT AT THE DOCTOR

In most cases, your first health care stop will be your primary care provider (PCP). If you're twenty-one or younger, that PCP might be your pediatrician (many see patients until they're out of college). If you've moved on from the doctor you went to when you were a kid, you probably have what's called a *GP* or *general practitioner*. You might also refer to that doctor as a *family doctor* or *internist* (they're all technically a little different but serve the same general purpose). PCPs are great at providing routine care: giving you immunizations when you need them, prescribing an antibiotic for an ear infection, or stitching up a small wound. But when you're having a chronic or long-term issue with a specific part of your body, it usually makes sense to see a specialist who's an expert in that one area to help you get to the bottom of things. In the case of stomach issues, that specialist is called a *gastroenterologist*, casually referred to as a *GI doc*.

Depending on how your family's health insurance works, you may have to see your PCP before you can visit a gastroenterologist to get what's called a referral (basically a permission slip to see any specialist, in this case the GI doc). Even if your insurance doesn't require a referral before you can see a gastroenterologist, it might be good to see your PCP to get a recommendation for a gut doctor she trusts. Your PCP may also know of a pediatric gastroenterologist, who specializes in young people's gut issues, or one who has a lot of experience with teens in your area.

When you see a gastroenterologist, the appointment will start out very much like an appointment with your general practitioner. You'll likely fill out a medical history form, giving the details of your health, lifestyle, and symptoms. Either you can fill this out or your parent can do it for you—it really depends on what feels most comfortable, although I recommend that you do it yourself with a little help as needed on things like whether there's any history of colon polyps in your family or whether you've ever had a bad reaction from a medication. The reason: You are the one with the symptoms, and only you know what you're truly going through. Also, before you know it—in college, maybe after—you'll find yourself at a doctor's office without a parent on hand to ask for support. So now's the best time to learn, with someone who cares about you there to show you the ropes.

Your gastroenterologist will likely run a number of tests, depending on your symptoms and what she thinks the problem might be. They may not all happen that day, though—some tests require a prescription to go to a testing facility; others may need you to prepare beforehand by eating or avoiding certain foods or discontinuing medication you're currently on.

In the paragraphs that follow, I've explained the tests your gastroenterologist might ask you to get up close and personal with; you won't have to have all of these tests, but rather one or a few that your doctor narrows it down to, depending on your specific symptoms and medical history. (Some of the ones I've listed here, a doctor might be less likely to ask a younger person to have, but I've included them just in case). Your doctor may also recommend that you have a test that's not on this list; it's near impossible for me to include every diagnostic procedure that's out there, and with constantly evolving technology there's no way of knowing what might be available in the future (not to mention, different doctors and labs don't always use the same tests). Here are some of the tests that you may hear about and should have on your radar.

## Oh, the Tests You'll Get!*

Blood test: Few people like having their blood drawn. But it's worth the mild discomfort of a needle to uncover the wealth of information you can

*Not all of these, I promise.

find from a simple blood test. Your doctor may look for the *HLA-DQ2* and *HLA-DQ8* genes—the indicators that show you are at risk for celiac disease. Depending on blood test results, your doctor may also determine that you have anemia, or markers of inflammation like a high white blood cell count or C-reactive protein score, which will help him find clues that can lead to a diagnosis. Your doctor might also have other levels checked, like thyroid hormones and vitamin D, which might help put some of the pieces of your health puzzle together.

**Stool analysis:** Ick. I know. But bear with me. One benefit of testing your stool—a.k.a. *poop*—is that your doctor will look for harmful parasites and their eggs that could be causing uncomfortable digestive symptoms. While I truly hope that none of those little nasty bugs have invaded your insides, here's the good news: If you have one, your doctor may be able to prescribe medication to make it go away, and cure your symptoms like that (I'm snapping my fingers). Your doctor will also be looking for things like blood in the stool as well as abnormal amounts of fat, both markers

of intestinal damage that can help narrow down what the problem might be. So how, you may be wondering, do you submit a stool sample? Well, I'm so glad you asked. Your doctor will likely give you a stool sample kit with a plastic hat-shaped bowl to place on your toilet. The indented part of this fancy hat that you'll *never, ever* want to put on your head fits right inside the toilet seat above the water so it catches the poop when you go. Your kit will also come with little plastic spoons or shovels and small, sterile vials to scoop samples into. Fun? No. Necessary? Yes, if your doctor says so. My tip: This, too, shall pass. Put on your "I can do anything once" hat (er, maybe something else), do it as quickly as possible, and then wash your hands— well. Laugh. You're tough as crap, and you're tougher than crap (too much?). The end.

**Lactose breath test:** This procedure requires you to drink a beverage that is high in lactose, a sugar found in milk and other dairy foods. Your doctor will then have you breathe into a plastic bag so he can measure the amount of hydrogen you are expelling. The reason: If your body doesn't process lactose (as a result of not producing enough lactase, the enzyme that breaks down lactose), the un-broken-down sugar will continue moving along the digestive tract until it reaches the large intestine. The very hungry bacteria in your large intestine see the lactose and think, "Mmm, lunch!" They then feed on (technical term: *ferment*) the lactose, resulting in the production of gases, including hydrogen. This test will take roughly three hours. You'll likely need to not eat for several hours and avoid certain foods and medications in the days and weeks before the test; talk to your doctor or clinic for details.

Fructose intolerance breath test: This procedure is very similar to a lactose intolerance breath test, however, the solution you drink contains fructose, a sugar found in foods like honey, apples, and mangoes. You eat a high-fructose food, then breathe into a bag that your doctor checks for a high percentage of hydrogen to indicate whether your body is digesting the fructose the way it should be or fermenting it, undigested, in the large intestine, causing uncomfortable symptoms like gas and diarrhea. The test will take around three hours and will also require you not to eat just

before it and to avoid certain foods and medications in the days leading up to it.

SIBO breath test (such as a glucose breath test or lactulose breath test): Normally, the bacteria in your large intestine ferment carbohydrates to produce the gases methane and hydrogen. In the condition known as small intestinal bacterial overgrowth (SIBO), the bacteria that should be found in the large intestine have pushed their way into an area that's not meant to handle so much bacteria—the small intestine. Think of them as your perfectly fine next-door neighbors who brought their sleeping bags and pillows over and made themselves at home in your living room, eating all of the groceries before your mom gets them into the kitchen. This hungry bacteria-where-it-doesn't-belong problem, called *SIBO*, is linked with a long list of problems like nutrient malabsorption (your body not being able to use vitamins and minerals the way it's supposed to), diarrhea, and more (I talk more about this condition on page 37). To test for SIBO, your doctor will have you drink a solution with a form of sugar in it. Then, every fifteen minutes you'll breathe into a bag, the contents of which will be analyzed for the gases methane and/or hydrogen. Depending on how much and how quickly the methane and/or hydrogen levels rise, your doctor can determine if you have an excess of bacteria in your small intestine (a.k.a. SIBO) and, as a result, the best way to treat you. This test will take at least two hours—which is annoying, but totally better than some house crashers taking your Cheetos.

**Upper endoscopy:** In this procedure, your doctor will send a thin, flexible tube called an endoscope down your throat into the upper part of your digestive tract—the esophagus, stomach, and duodenum. Using the miniscule camera at the end of the tube, your doctor can look at images of your upper digestive lining on a video monitor; she can also take tissue samples or biopsies to test for various conditions. You will likely be sedated for this test; if nothing else the doctor will spray your throat with an anesthetic so discomfort is kept to a minimum. You won't be allowed to eat in the hours leading up to the test.

**Capsule endoscopy:** This test sounds like something out of some futuristic reality show gone bad. Before you've eaten in the morning, you swallow a pill-like capsule that has a camera in it. The camera takes pictures as it makes its way through the gastrointestinal tract; you'll wear a belt around your waist that helps record the photos while you go about your business for eight hours or so. This test makes it easier for doctors to see inside the small intestine, which can be hard to reach via traditional endoscopy. As for what happens to the teeny-tiny camera? It will come out in your poop. It is safe to flush it down the toilet, so don't gross yourself out trying to find it (you're welcome).

**Balloon-assisted enteroscopy:** You will be sedated for this procedure, in which your doctor sends a long tube with one or two balloons into your small intestine. By inflating and deflating the balloon, the doctor makes the scope grip the walls of the intestine and inch its way deep into the twenty-foot-long organ to see what's going on. Because this is an invasive procedure, it would likely be done only after other tests proved inadequate.

**Colonoscopy:** Ah, everyone's favorite (#sarcasm)—not just because of the procedure itself, but because of the

# Enema of the State

If someone mentions getting an enema, don't freak out. Enemas are weird, sure, but no weirder than any of the rest of the symptoms you've been going through. Here's what it entails: Using a tube, someone injects fluid through your rectum. The result is basically insta-laxative—in other words, the pressure from the added liquid kicks your colon into high gear, and after a few minutes anything and everything that's in there gets sent right out into the toilet. Your doctor may suggest using it to relieve constipation, or as a clean-out before a procedure.

lengthy prep that anyone who gets one is required to do before the test. Since most adults routinely start getting colonoscopies at age fifty—younger if they have an increased risk for colon cancer—you may have heard about this one from a grandparent, parent, or older friend who has gone through it. A colonoscopy, as given away by the name, looks for abnormalities in the colon, which as you know (because you read Chapter 1 so closely) is another name for the large intestine—the cavity in which water is absorbed and poop goes from a liquid to a semisolid state. In order for your doctor to get a good look at the colon, it needs to be empty. Hence the clean-out-your-colon precolonoscopy prep. If your doctor decides this is the right test for you, he'll ask you to get ready by chugging a special drink or taking medication the day before the test to ensure your colon is poop-free (your doctor will give you specific instructions regarding the prep method he uses; you will also be required to stop taking certain medications and eating specific foods in the days leading up to it). Your doctor will also ask you to eat only clear liquids the day before the test, because what goes in must come out (Jell-O, Popsicles, and Gatorade are usually OK; check with your doctor for specifics). If you're doing a colonoscopy prep, the most important two words you can hear are these: *Stay home.* You will have to go to the bathroom—a lot. Often urgently. Stay near a toilet. Some people recommend keeping wet wipes or baby wipes on hand to prevent your tush from getting sore. Pick out a few movies you've wanted to watch on Netflix, take it easy, and relax as much as you can.

As for the actual test itself: The visit can take three to four hours from start to finish, though the procedure itself won't last for more than an hour. You will likely be sedated, which is why most clinics require you have someone present to safely drive you home afterward. During the test, you'll wear a hospital gown and lie on your side while the doctor passes a scope through your rear end up into your now empty colon (you'll be glad you went through all of that spring cleaning the day before). He'll examine the lining of the colon and may use another instrument to take a sample of the lining for analysis. Your doctor will probably be able to discuss the results with you when you're finished, though you'll have to wait for a lab to analyze any samples taken. And that's that. Give yourself a pat on the back. You've completed something many people have to wait until their fifties to experience. And now it's over. You rock.

**Flexible sigmoidoscopy:** This test looks at the rectum and lower (a.k.a. *sigmoid*) colon using a bendable tube that has a light and a small camera at the end of it to give your doctor the ability to take a closer look at that portion of the GI tract. The prep for a flexible sigmoidoscopy is similar to that for a colonoscopy, for the same reasons. This procedure is shorter and less involved than a colonoscopy, though, which is why your doctor is less likely to sedate you for this one. You'll lie on the table

## How Can I Take My Mind Off My Test?

Comfort is not the first thing that comes to mind when someone says a word like *colonoscopy* or *endoscopy*, or anything that ends in *-oscopy*, come to think of it. So helping you feel as calm, cool, and collected as possible during any procedure you might have is one of my big goals. My top tip: Ask your doctor what you will be allowed to do and come prepared. Are smartphones allowed? Tablets? If so, have some podcasts, funny TV shows, or distracting music ready to go. If not, think out of the technology box. A book of crossword puzzles or a grown-up coloring book (or that Disney princess one you were quietly eyeing—it's OK, I love Ariel, too) can work wonders to keep your mind elsewhere.

on your side wearing a hospital gown so the doctor can insert the sigmoidoscope into your bottom. Take deep breaths, think about a happy place like the beach on a warm day with your best friends and know it will be over soon—twenty minutes or so, around the same time it takes to watch an episode of *Parks and Rec*, without the commercials.

**Anal manometry:** Remember those sphincter muscles that control the movement of poop into different parts of the GI tract, and finally out of your body (see pages 7 to 9)? This test measures how well the anal sphincter is working by inserting a small, flexible tube with a balloon on the end into the rectum while you lie on your side wearing a hospital gown (for similar reasons to the colonoscopy, the doctor will ask you to empty your bowels with an enema or other prep before the test). The tech will inflate and deflate the balloon to assess how well the muscles work. He may also ask you to squeeze, as if you're holding in a poop, or push, as if you're trying to get rid of one. The whole thing will take up to an hour.

**Gastric emptying scan (GES):** This test looks at how quickly your stomach contracts and moves food into your intestines. After fasting for six hours, you'll go to a testing center and eat a meal that contains radioactive material (don't try this at home!). After you've eaten, the technician will ask you to lie on your back while he uses something called a gamma camera to take pictures of your stomach. Have a few good podcasts cued up, because the tech will ask you to wait around so he can take more pictures at various intervals for several hours after the meal. What you can't do, however, is eat or drink anything else until the test is over.

**Upper GI and small bowel series:** This refers to a series of x-rays taken to get a closer look at the esophagus, stomach, and small intestine. Your doctor may give you an injection to slow the movement of muscles in the GI tract to make it easier for them to see what's going on. Before you go to the x-ray machine, your doctor will ask you to drink a beverage that tastes something like a milk shake; it contains barium, which makes it easier to read the x-ray. The technician will ask you to sit or stand in various positions while he takes images that will give him a picture of what's going on in your insides. From start to finish, this test will take between three and six hours, so get those

## GETTING TESTED

"Stay calm and be open-minded."

"Try to go in relaxed."

"It's easy to worry about the worst possible outcome, but the fact you're getting help means you're even closer to getting treatment!"

"Remember that any procedure would be less uncomfortable and scary than having ongoing mysterious symptoms!"

"Just keep in mind that this is a temporary phase of life and it will pass."

podcasts queued up. You will likely have to change your diet or fast before the test, so talk to your doctor for details.

**Magnetic resonance enterography (MRE):** This test is a specific type of magnetic resonance imaging (MRI) that allows your doctor to take pictures of your small intestine using a magnetic field; some medical professionals prefer it to an x-ray, particularly for younger patients, because there's no radiation involved. The procedure can be noisy, so you may want to bring earplugs. After you arrive, you'll change into a gown; the doctor may give you a sedative to help you relax. You will drink a contrast fluid solution that will help the doctor

see your small intestine in the pictures; about forty-five minutes later the nurse will help you lay on an exam table, where the machine will scan your body. The technician may give you more contrast fluid or water through an IV. Afterward, you may feel some stomach upset from the contrast material; if it persists, let your doctor know. Because you will have been sedated, make sure an adult accompanies you to this procedure to drive you home (also to offer support!).

# DRUMROLL, PLEASE: A DIAGNOSIS

Once you've gone through the appropriate testing, it's the moment

## Health Insurance Hassles

Sadly, your health insurance plan may not cover all of the important tests your doctor recommends. The back of your health insurance ID card should have an 800 number on it that you can call for help; it's probably wise to give them a buzz (or have your parent do so) before any specialist visits or procedures to find out what's covered or if there's anything for which you'll need prior authorization, so your family doesn't get saddled with any surprise bills down the road. Your parent may also want to contact her HR representative for help.

you've been waiting for—your diagnosis. Or, in other words, the doctor finally tells you what she thinks is going on with your insides.

Gastrointestinal symptoms can be caused by any number of conditions. If we're going by the numbers, you're more likely to have irritable bowel syndrome (IBS) than any other digestive problem—but you may have IBD or another disorder. IBD stands for *inflammatory bowel disease* and is the shorthand medical pros use when referring most often to Crohn's disease and colitis (more on them in just a minute). Or instead of (or in addition to) these conditions, you may have something like celiac disease, lactose intolerance, or fructose malabsorption. Here's what you need to know about these and the other most common gut disorders you're likely to

hear come out of your doctor's mouth on diagnosis day.

## Irritable Bowel Syndrome (IBS)

Symptoms of IBS—one of the most common disorders of any type that causes people to visit their doctors— affects roughly one in every six or seven American teenagers and adults, so if you don't have IBS yourself, you almost undoubtedly know someone who does, even if he hasn't mentioned it in conversation.

Symptoms: So what's going on in the digestive tracts of the oh-so-many people who have IBS? Visibly, nothing—which is one major clue that can help doctors separate IBS from other digestive conditions. IBS is

# WHAT IT'S LIKE TO HAVE A GUT DISORDER

"I feel like shit all the time. It's ruining my life."

"It's painful and inconvenient."

"It's embarrassing, tiring, stressful, dreadful, painful."

"It's disruptive to my everyday life."

considered a functional gut disorder. In other words, your GI tract looks normal, but symptoms are sending you the message loud and clear that something isn't functioning (as in "functional gut disorder") as it should. It's actually considered a syndrome, or a group of symptoms, more than a disease. Doctors now believe that IBS and other functional GI disorders occur when your brain and gut aren't communicating as well as they should be.

IBS can look very different depending on the person who has it. Abdominal pain combined with changes in the frequency and consistency of your poop are the hallmark symptoms of IBS. In diarrhea-predominant IBS (also known as IBS-D) a person has frequent loose stools; with constipation-predominant IBS (also known as IBS-C), a person has a hard time going and has to do so

infrequently. A person with mixed IBS (IBS-M) alternates between the two.

Up until recently, IBS was a problem that was often experienced, but not frequently discussed. However, people's comfort levels with conversations about IBS seem to be increasing. A pricey TV commercial that aired during the 2016 Super Bowl advertising Xifaxan, an antibiotic used in the treatment of IBS, is a good example. Memorably starring a walking, talking, knotted-up intestine, it had people affectionately referring to the game as the "Super Bowel" for weeks. Probiotics have also started getting people talking about IBS more. These good-for-you, gut-balancing bugs are found in fermented foods like yogurt and sauerkraut as well as in pills that now make up one of the most popular dietary supplement categories in America and have sparked loads of chatter online, in magazines, and elsewhere about IBS and related issues. The once-unspoken disease is also landing on the pages of some of the most widely read magazines and websites thanks to the low-FODMAP diet, a plan designed by researchers specifically to help people minimize symptoms of IBS, and what this book is all about.

If you ask me, it's about time IBS stopped getting swept under the rug. Even though for people with IBS, the long-term repercussions of the disease aren't as grave as for some other digestive disorders (thankfully) and the symptoms may not always be as dramatic as some other gut diseases, what is serious is the toll it can take on people's well-being. IBS can severely diminish a person's quality of life—in other words, how well you can go about your daily routines and simply live the way you want to live. Research has found that quality of life is worse for people with IBS than for those with other also-potentially debilitating conditions like asthma, migraines, and acid reflux. About 68 percent of people with IBS report that they miss at least ten activities during a three-month span because of their symptoms; more than half say that IBS has had a significant impact on their social lives.

**Who gets it:** Around the world, IBS affects anywhere between 10 and 35 percent of people, and race/ethnicity doesn't seem to play a major role. A person can develop the disease at any age, although doctors seem to diagnose it less in older patients. According to Dr. Brian Lacy in his book *Making Sense of IBS*, most adults with IBS began to develop symptoms in their late teenage years or early twenties (it's possible for it to begin earlier or later); so if you're a young person who has been diagnosed with IBS, you're certainly not alone. Many who experience symptoms at a young age, however, won't be diagnosed for years to come. In other words, by getting a diagnosis now and figuring out how you can best manage the condition, you may be saving yourself years of discomfort and trouble, not to mention unwanted time off from school and work. Go. You.

While both males and females can develop IBS, women are more likely to be diagnosed with the syndrome than men. This may be due to hormonal fluctuations, which can worsen symptoms, but may also be in part due to women being more likely to visit with their doctor for routine care, opening up an opportunity for a doctor to take notice of anything that sounds off.

So what causes IBS to interfere in *your* life and not the lives of the other six kids in your study hall? There are a number of factors that may contribute to the disease's development, it seems; there's no one cause or chain of events that are responsible for the high levels of IBS throughout the world. Here are some potential puzzle pieces that may be working in tandem, resulting in IBS and IBS-like symptoms:

- *Genetics:* Having family members— particularly first-degree ones like a mother, father, brother, or sister—with IBS may make you more inclined to develop it yourself. (But it's important to remember that although a genetic predisposition passed down by your parents may increase your chances of having IBS at some point, it is not a given that you'll get it. )

- *Gut-brain miscommunication:* Have you ever had a "gut feeling" about

something, or had someone tell you upon being faced with a tough decision to "go with your gut"? There's a reason why these phrases exist, and experts actually refer to your digestive tract as your "second brain" because its lining is covered with more than a hundred million nerve cells that gather information and communicate back and forth with your OG brain. Doctors still have a lot to learn about this link, but they now know that the way in which these two "brains" talk to each other may be at the core of many people's struggles with IBS.

- *Wonky bacteria:* Teeny-tiny microbes are a crucial part of your body, particularly in your digestive tract. But an imbalance of those little bugs— either too many of certain kinds, not enough of others, or their growth in the wrong places—may set the stage for IBS to develop, as well as cause specific symptoms.

- *Messed-up movements:* Sometimes the digestive tract of someone with IBS looks like the worst contestants on *Dancing with the Stars*—totally uncoordinated but trying really, really hard. Under healthy circumstances, this stretching and contracting of the muscles lining the GI tract helps push food on its digestive journey. When those movements, known as gastrointestinal motility, go awry, it can lead to various symptoms of IBS.

- *Supersensitivity:* Has anyone ever told you you're a little bit oversensitive? Well, if you have IBS that might be true (in the case of IBS, though, it's technically called *visceral hypersensitivity*). Research shows that some people with IBS experience gut pain more intensely than those without IBS. In other words, if you have more sensitive nerve endings in your gut, you experience more pain and discomfort in it than a less-sensitive person does when, for instance, an imbalance of bacteria in the colon creates extra gas (see how all of these factors might be working together?).

- *Holey intestines:* Increased intestinal permeability, sometimes referred to as a "leaky gut," is the idea that the layer of mucosal tissue that lines the intestines to protect the body from invasion by bad guys (like microorganisms) gets a little too lenient. These tissues are supposed to allow fluids and nutrients to pass through, but if you have leaky gut, they also let in things they shouldn't, which get absorbed into your bloodstream and go right ahead and make themselves at home. The body senses foreign invaders, resulting in an autoimmune response, which can cause many symptoms, including digestive ones.

- *Other digestive conditions:* The symptoms of digestive conditions such as lactose intolerance, fructose intolerance, SIBO, celiac disease, Crohn's disease, ulcerative colitis, and more can overlap immensely with the symptoms of IBS—so much so that it may be difficult to separate them. If you are being treated for another digestive disorder but still have IBS-like symptoms, talk to your doctor about incorporating treatment for IBS, like a low-FODMAP diet, into your current treatment.

How is it treated: How IBS is treated depends on your symptoms and your doctor and you. There is, unfortunately, no one-size-fits-all treatment for IBS. Up until pretty recently, doctors were somewhat limited in terms of treatment options to offer patients diagnosed with the disease. Nowadays, things seem to be changing. There are several prescription medications, probiotic supplements, and herbal remedies your doctor may want you to try. And stress management through exercise as well as meditation can also help (see Chapter 8). What's more, the groundbreaking low-FODMAP diet—a plan that minimizes specific carbohydrates that are not digested well and can lead to gas-producing fermentation in the gut as well as pull water into the GI tract—is giving us a valuable and highly effective tool to help people manage their IBS. The next chapters will introduce you to the low-FODMAP plan and tell you how to make it fit into your busy life.

## Crohn's Disease

Crohn's disease is an inflammatory bowel disease (IBD). An IBD is different from IBS in that it signifies chronic inflammation, damage to the intestines, and an inappropriate immune response. Crohn's can cause damage anywhere along the lining of the GI tract, from the mouth to the anus—but it most

commonly affects the end of the small bowel (or ileum) and the beginning of the colon. It can also affect the entire thickness of the bowel wall.

**Symptoms:** Persistent diarrhea, rectal bleeding, an urgent need to move your bowels, abdominal cramps, the sensation that you are still going or still need to go after you've just gone, constipation, fever, loss of appetite, and/ or weight loss

**Who gets it:** Around 0.2 percent of the population has Crohn's disease. Crohn's tends to run in families, so if you have a relative with it, you may be more likely to develop it yourself. It's most common in people with eastern European backgrounds, though in recent years it's increased among African Americans as well. It's also more common in urban environments and in northern rather than southern climates.

**How it's treated:** Crohn's is usually treated with medication that will tell your overactive immune system to take it easy; once your immune system calms down, inflammation will decrease and your gut can actually heal. Your doctor will weigh the benefits and risks of several prescriptions that are used. Diets like the specific carbohydrate diet (SCD; see page 49) and the low-FODMAP plan (see, well, the rest of this book) may also help you manage symptoms. Talk to your medical team about what you might try (and keep reading for more on how food can help).

## Ulcerative Colitis

In ulcerative colitis, an inflammatory bowel disease, the lining of the colon becomes inflamed and develops sores—called ulcers—that produce mucus and pus. This abnormal response is a result of your immune system malfunctioning; it mistakes materials in your intestine for foreign invaders, so your body sends white blood cells to the intestinal lining, which produces inflammation and damage. Ulcerative colitis is different

from Crohn's disease in that it only affects the innermost lining of the colon.

**Symptoms:** Loose and urgent bowel movements, persistent and painful diarrhea, blood in your stool, crampy abdominal pain, loss of appetite, and/or weight loss

**Who gets it:** Around 0.2 percent of the population is affected by ulcerative colitis. It tends to run in families and is more common among people of eastern European descent and those who are Jewish. Men and women are equally likely to be affected, and while it can occur at any age, most people with the disease are diagnosed in their midthirties.

**How it's treated:** Your doctor may put you on one or more medications

## Montezuma's Revenge Times a Million

Research is uncovering the links between short-term bouts of belly sickness—like you would experience from the flu or traveler's diarrhea—and IBS. It seems that even a quickie bug may have the potential to injure or alter the GI tract in a way that causes some people to develop IBS. If you think back to when you first started to notice symptoms that just wouldn't go away, you very well may be able to connect it with a few unpleasant days you spent losing your lunch. Ah, the gift that keeps on giving.

Of course, while IBS affects more people than any other gut disorder, there are still plenty of us out there with other conditions—and several that may have some overlap with IBS and its symptoms. In this section, I introduce you to some other disorders your doctor may uncover.

to suppress inflammation and allow your gut to heal. As many as one third of people with ulcerative colitis will eventually require surgery to remove the colon. Diet can also play a role— again, eating plans like the SCD and low-FODMAP may give you additional relief. Talk with your health care team to develop the best plan for you.

## Celiac Disease

Celiac disease is an autoimmune disorder that causes the body to attack itself when a person eats gluten, a protein found in wheat, rye, and barley. This leads to damage in the small intestine that can flatten the villi (see page 7) and diminish nutrient absorption. If celiac disease isn't treated, the impact over time can lead to serious health problems.

Symptoms: Diarrhea, constipation, anemia, joint pain, itchy skin rashes, headaches, ADHD, short stature, and/or delayed growth or puberty

Who gets it: Around 1 percent of the US population has celiac disease. It runs in families—if you have a parent or sibling with it you have a one-in-ten chance of developing the disease.

How it's treated: The only way to treat celiac disease is by adhering to a strict gluten-free diet for life, avoiding not

## AVOIDING BATHROOM ACCIDENTS

"Always make sure you know where you're going and where the closest bathroom is and have some air freshener or some sort of spray with you."

"Make sure you have spare underwear and pants with you at all times."

"It sounds funny, but . . . squeeze your butt shut and think about something else until you reach the bathroom!"

just the protein itself but also potential sources of cross-contamination (even crumbs from a toaster or deep fryer can be damaging). Since there may be some overlap with IBS, a person with celiac who is strictly gluten-free but still experiencing symptoms may want to try out the low-FODMAP plan in addition to their very necessary gluten-free one. See a registered dietitian nutritionist first to make sure you aren't eating any surprise sources of gluten and to get some guidance on what to try next.

## Lactose Intolerance

People with lactose intolerance don't produce enough of the enzyme lactase, which breaks down lactose, a sugar in milk and other dairy products. As a result, undigested lactose passes into the colon, where bacteria feed on it, creating fluid and gas.

Symptoms: Abdominal bloating, abdominal pain, diarrhea, gas, and/or nausea—all of which occur thirty minutes to two hours after consuming milk or dairy products

Who gets it: Lactose intolerance affects 65 percent of humans across the world. Blacks, Hispanics/Latinos, American Indians, and people of Asian descent are more likely to have lactose intolerance than those of northern European descent. It's also common in people of West African, Arab, Jewish, Greek, and Italian descent. People who suffer from lactose intolerance frequently also suffer from IBS (and vice versa).

## OMG, I CAN'T BELIEVE THIS HAPPENED.

"One time my stomach made a loud noise in math, and someone behind me said to the person beside him, 'I just heard her stomach make a noise.' Let me just say, my face was *so* red."

"I was at my boyfriend's house and had to go home desperately, and he thought I didn't want to be with him anymore because I didn't tell him I needed to poo."

"I was with my friend at a restaurant eating food that was labeled 'gluten-free,' but I knew it wasn't after I ate it. When I went back to her house to use the bathroom, I was in and out of it for probably two hours."

"I spent around twenty minutes in the toilet and did a number two. When I walked out, there was a lady who just looked down at me and said, "That was long." I honestly didn't know what to say."

**How it's treated:** Depending on the level of severity, it's treated either by avoiding lactose altogether or by eating it only in small amounts as tolerated, consuming lactose-free dairy products, and/or taking lactase enzyme pills any time you eat a milk-containing food.

## Fructose Malabsorption or Intolerance

Everyone can digest only so much fructose, the sugar found in fruits and some vegetables, honey, agave, as well as packaged foods like sports drinks, soda, and candy made with high-fructose corn syrup. A person with fructose malabsorption (sometimes also referred to as *fructose intolerance* or *dietary fructose intolerance*), however, is even more sensitive. As a result, fructose passes through the GI tract and lands in the large intestines, where bacteria are all too happy to eat it up, produce gas, and cause digestive distress. A person with fructose malabsorption might also have problems with fructans, chains of fructose found in foods like wheat, garlic, and onions. ***Note:*** Fructose is best absorbed alongside another sugar, glucose. Foods that contain a too-big proportion of fructose relative to glucose are the ones most likely to give a person with fructose malabsorption problems. Fructose malabsorption may be related to the symptoms of IBS; following a low-FODMAP diet may help you feel better if you are sensitive to this carbohydrate, as well as pinpoint any others you may be having trouble with. You may also want to talk to a registered dietitian nutritionist specifically about how to avoid foods with a high proportion of fructose.

**Symptoms:** Gas, bloating, diarrhea, and abdominal pain

**Who gets it:** Anyone. Ethnicity doesn't seem to be a factor in how likely you are to experience fructose malabsorption; some research finds that it may be more common in children and may decrease with age, although that has not been found consistently. As much as half the population is unable to tolerate 25 grams of fructose, roughly the amount found in one soda.

**How it's treated:** It's treated by avoiding high amounts of excess fructose, or fructose that's not balanced with glucose, at one time.

## Small Intestinal Bacterial Overgrowth (SIBO)

As mentioned on page 21, SIBO is a condition in which bacteria that should be living in the colon spread out and take over space in the small intestine, where they don't belong. I compared it to when your perfectly nice next-door neighbors decide to move in. Experts suggest that SIBO may occur due to an inadequately activated *migrating motor complex* (see page 9); in other words, that "clean-sweep" wave isn't happening as often as it needs to.

**Symptoms:** Bloating, gas, diarrhea, and/or constipation

**Who gets it:** SIBO may have a close connection with IBS; one study linked it with as many as 84 percent of IBS cases (20 percent of healthy volunteers also tested positive!). Other research, however, has linked it with 10 percent of IBS patients. It's also possible for SIBO to be present in people who have celiac disease, IBD, and other gut disorders; an increased risk is also shown for those who have diabetes, people who frequently use antibiotics, and those with low stomach acid, among other conditions. It may also be more common in older patients compared with younger people.

How it's treated: Currently, doctors primarily treat SIBO with antibiotics; at the moment there is no evidence-based diet recommended, though people do use the low-FODMAP plan along with several others outlined in this book.

One important note about SIBO and food, however: If you're being treated with antibiotics, don't even think about trying a special diet like low-FODMAP until you're done with your prescription and the doctor says it's OK. A low-FODMAP plan essentially limits the food the bugs thrive on, which sends them into hibernation. If you don't feed the bugs, then they won't be out and about for the antibiotics to take care of.

# CHAPTER 3

# But What should I Eat?

## THE LOW-FODMAP PLAN AND OTHER DIET OPTIONS

So you've been to the doctor and spilled your guts about, well, your guts. And maybe you've even been lucky enough to run through the gamut of testing, from blood work to stool study to upper endoscopy to everyone's favorite test, the colonoscopy (we know, your friends are jealous). And at the end of the medical marathon, your doctor has—I sincerely hope—been able to give you an answer about what's ailing you.

## THE GUT-FOOD CONNECTION

What comes next depends very much on your doctor and the condition that you've been diagnosed with. Medication may be part of your treatment plan, and so might dietary supplements like probiotics (see Chapter 7), as well as stress-management techniques (see Chapter 8). The other crucial component

that (shockingly!) doesn't always get the attention it deserves is diet. Think about it—you have a disease that affects the parts of your body that digest and process food. Of course food plays a role in your illness! Of the teens I surveyed as I was writing this book, around half said that their doctors addressed their diets, some suggesting a specific plan and others suggesting that patients give some consideration to foods that might

# WHY I TRIED LOW FODMAPS

"My doctor suggested a low-FODMAP diet."

"My doctor suggested that I make a diary of what made my symptoms worse. I then found out about the FODMAP diet online and decided to give it a go."

"My mom, who is a dietitian, thought it might help."

be related to increases in symptoms. I was so glad to hear that.

The other half of teens that I surveyed, however, said that their doctors never brought up the topic of what to eat. This is a huge problem. Food choices can play a major role in your healing from and control of digestive issues like IBS, Crohn's, ulcerative colitis, celiac disease, and more (to be fair, since going on a 100 percent gluten-free diet is only way to manage celiac disease, doctors are wonderful at prescribing a gluten-free diet for that condition, although some people with celiac may require an extra step beyond going gluten-free, which is an often missed detail). What's more, going on a special diet doesn't have a steep price tag, aside from the normal costs associated with food, and won't surprise you with hidden side effects. Diet is not everything, true, and there are plenty of times when other measures are called for. But changing the way you eat as part of your treatment plan can be a crucial part of digestive disease management—and for many people, diet alone can keep symptoms under control.

Some GI doctors are very diet literate and may suggest a specific eating plan and even refer you to a registered dietitian nutritionist to help you get started. Other doctors, however, are not as clued in to how much food can affect your symptoms. In my work as a registered dietitian nutritionist, I've seen too many clients with gastrointestinal disorders overwhelmed when it comes to how to eat. Between blogs, BuzzFeed, and Aunt Bertha (who wants nothing more than to corner you at Thanksgiving and tell you what helped her get rid of unbearable gas, again), there's a ton of information out there about eating to improve gut problems. If you're feeling confused, you're not alone. My goal in this chapter is to separate fact from fiction, science from nonsense, and rumor from reality about the various diets that people tend to go on for GI issues. I also want to make sure you know about a research-backed diet that is extremely effective in treating IBS and can also help people with other gut disorders: the low-FODMAP plan.

## GETTING TO KNOW LOW FODMAPS

When I learned of the low-FODMAP diet for treatment of irritable bowel syndrome, I was floored. A diet that could improve or even eliminate the symptoms of IBS, a condition that often leaves people in pain and frustrated and for which there is no standard, reliable treatment? In my work as a registered dietitian nutritionist, I'd seen so many clients suffering with IBS who had few strategies to help them manage their symptoms. The first time I suggested low FODMAPs to an IBS client, I was working with a young lady who lived on a perfectly healthy but high-in-

FODMAP diet of bread, hummus, and apples. When I saw how her symptoms were reversed—reversed!—with dietary changes alone, I was sold. I've continued to recommend the low-FODMAP plan to clients (and friends and family!) with much success.

I later learned that a low-FODMAP plan might also help people with other gut disorders manage their symptoms. I stopped in my tracks. I needed to know more. And so do you. Here are the basics:

Since the early 2000s, researchers in Australia have uncovered some clues about what might be contributing to the symptoms of IBS. Their research led them to develop a diet called *low-FODMAP*, which successfully treats unpleasant effects like gas, bloating, diarrhea, and constipation by altering a person's eating habits. In recent years, the plan has begun to gain some well-deserved attention throughout the rest of the world, including the United States; if you've never heard of it, prepare yourself—it's about to become a lot more well known. It may also change your life.

### What's the Plan?

*FODMAP* is an acronym that refers to carbohydrates commonly found in our diets. The letters stand for "fermentable oligo-, di-, monosaccharides and polyols." A mouthful, yes—which is why we'll stick with *FODMAP*. What sets FODMAP carbohydrates apart from others is that the small intestine, in some people, has a harder time digesting them. As a result, these undigested carbohydrates stay on the digestion train and get transported into the large intestine (a.k.a. *colon*), where bacteria ferment them, which produces gases; they also have a tendency to pull in excess fluid. Most people, it seems, aren't great at digesting FODMAPs, but that often doesn't cause any real harm to their systems, and they feel just fine. For a good many others, though, that fermentation in the large intestine causes painful gas, bloating, diarrhea, and other uncomfortable symptoms.

The big picture of the low-FODMAP plan is pretty straightforward: By limiting the amount of FODMAPs in the diet, the amount of fermentation and fluid in the colon is lessened, and therefore, so are the unpleasant symptoms that they cause in people with sensitive guts. When those Australian doctors first ran a pilot study to test their FODMAP hypothesis, they found that a low-FODMAP diet improved the symptoms of 74 percent of the sixty-two IBS and fructose malabsorption patients who followed

it. That seemed too good to be true—except in the years since, researchers have run several bigger and more thorough studies, and the results have been consistent: Roughly three out of four people with IBS who follow a low-FODMAP diet seem to reverse their symptoms.

What about those with inflammatory bowel diseases like Crohn's disease and ulcerative colitis? Well, for these people, the main goals are reversing inflammation and healing gut damage, and, depending on the severity of their condition, medication or even surgery may be necessary. But remember what we said in Chapter 2 about overlap? People with IBD also have a good chance of experiencing functional gut symptoms like gas, bloating, and diarrhea—those that may occur in IBS. In fact, 57 percent of patients with in-remission Crohn's disease and 33 percent of patients with in-remission ulcerative colitis—in other words, their inflammation was under control—had experienced IBS-like symptoms in the week before being surveyed by researchers in Sweden, according to one study published in the *American Journal of Gastroenterology*. Another study found that when people with IBD (both Crohn's and colitis) who experienced IBS-like symptoms went on a low-FODMAP diet, more than half felt an overall improvement. Those who had bloating, abdominal pain, and diarrhea were most likely to improve, while people with symptoms like constipation and nausea were less likely.

What about people with celiac disease? As many as 20 percent of people with the autoimmune response to gluten continue to have digestive symptoms while on a gluten-free diet, according to the Celiac Disease Foundation. This means that these unfortunate souls will have to go through the frustration of feeling unwell, getting a diagnosis, working hard to follow a restrictive diet in hopes of recovery, and still feeling tortured by their symptoms. There is, of course, the possibility that a person in this situation is still experiencing symptoms due to accidental gluten ingestion from unexpected sources like lip gloss or a "gluten-free" (but baked in a kitchen that used wheat flour) pizza. But again, there's also the chance for overlap—a person with celiac disease may also have IBS or another digestive disorder. If you're among the 20 percent of people with diagnosed celiac disease who isn't feeling better on a gluten-free diet, I urge you to see your doctor to explore the possibility that you might have another condition. And depending on the results of those tests, you, too, may benefit from a low-FODMAP plan.

To really understand what a low-FODMAP plan entails, you have to get to know the letters that make up the FODMAP acronym. Here's what each one means (brought to you in super-enthusiastic-cheerleader style because you're on the way to digestive health: V-I-C-T-O-R-Y!!!! Also, this section will start feeling like a chemistry textbook if I don't do something to add some E-N-E-R-G-Y!!!! Woooohoooo, go team!!!! Exclamation points for everyone!!!!).

## What to Avoid If Ya Got IBS? F-O-D-M-A-P-S!

Gimme an F! The *F* in *FODMAP* stands for *fermentable*. This applies to all of the carbohydrates you need to avoid in the FODMAP plan—the letters that come next are the different classes of carbohydrates you have to look out for.

Gimme an O! The *O* in *FODMAP* stands for *oligosaccharides*, which are carbohydrates made up of short chains of sugar molecules. There are two classes of fermentable oligosaccharides that we talk about when it comes to the low-FODMAP diet:

- Fructo-oligosaccharides (FOS), or fructans, are chains of fructose sugar molecules (also known as fruit sugar) strung together. They're found in wheat, rye, onions, garlic, and more.
- Galacto-oligosaccharides (GOS) are galactose sugar molecules strung together. They're found in certain legumes like black beans, kidney beans, baked beans, and peas.

Gimme a D! The *D* in *FODMAP* stands for **disaccharides**, which are carbohydrates made up of two sugar molecules fused together. Not all disaccharides may be fermented by people with sensitive guts, however. The one you need to know is lactose. Lactose is made up of the two simple sugars glucose and galactose. If it sounds familiar, that's because we talked about it on page 35 when we talked about lactose intolerance, or the inability to break down lactose due to having low levels of the enzyme lactase. Lactose is found only in dairy foods like milk, cheese, ice cream, and yogurt. But, low FODMAPs doesn't have to mean dairy-free. Many dairy foods are available in lactose-free versions (the manufacturers add some lactase enzyme, which breaks down the lactose for you). Plus, hard or ripened cheeses like Parmesan, cheddar,

and Gouda should only have minimal amounts of lactose in them. Fermented dairy foods like yogurt and kefir may also be tolerated by some with IBS because the fermentation process diminishes the amount of lactose in a food.

Gimme an M! The *M* in *FODMAP* stands for **monosaccharides**. If disaccharides are carbohydrates made of two sugar molecules fused together, then what do you think *monosaccharide* means? If you guessed one sugar molecule, you're absolutely right. The single sugar molecule that may be fermented in the gut is fructose, often referred to as "fruit sugar." Fructose is found in fruits and vegetables as well as honey and high-fructose corn syrup (a man-made sweetener used in packaged foods). It is interesting that fructose is only a problem for people who don't digest it well when it is more abundant than the amount of glucose (another simple sugar) in a food. Think of it this way: Glucose, which is easily digested, can take fructose by the hand and walk it across the lining of the intestine, so you absorb both without consequence. Fructose is a problem only when it's left all alone or when there's not enough glucose to help. The only way to know what foods contain excess fructose is to refer to a source that has gathered such information; I'll make it easy for you in Chapter 4. Some examples of foods with excess fructose are apples, mangos, watermelons, asparagus, sugar snap peas, honey, high-fructose corn syrup, and agave nectar.

**Gimme a P!** The *P* in *FODMAP* stands for *polyols*. Polyols are also known as sugar alcohols, though they're neither sugar nor alcoholic and can often be identified by the *-ol* at the end of them: mannitol, sorbitol, xylitol, and maltitol as well as polydextrose and isomalt. They can be found naturally, as in foods like blackberries, plums, cauliflower, and mushrooms; however, they also show up frequently in artificially sweetened sugar-free foods, like gums and mints.

**What does that spell?** *FODMAP!*

**And what do you wanna do?** *Limit the intake of them to prevent excess fermentation and extra water from being pulled into your gut and to eliminate your unpleasant gut symptoms.*

OK, so that last part of the cheer doesn't work that well. But what you really need to remember is easy enough—just don't eat too many FODMAPs. Except . . . there's really no way to tell what foods have a high level of FODMAPs by looking at them or even by thinking really hard about it. Fear not, my friend! In the next chapter, I'll make it easy for you to figure out what foods are OK to eat on a low-FODMAP plan and which ones you'll save for later. But first, we've got some ground to cover on the other eating plans you should know about.

## UNDERSTANDING THE GAGGLE OF GUT HEALTH DIETS

I'm a big advocate of the low-FODMAP plan, which I've seen help so many people; the science behind why it works makes a lot of sense, and the research testing how effective it can be is convincing. However, it's not the only food-based approach to managing GI symptoms. In fact, the low-FODMAP diet is actually one of the newer regimens on the gut health scene; there are a range of other food plans you may hear about from friends, close relatives, second cousins once removed, health professionals, complete strangers, and the Internet while on your journey to gut wellness.

Before you make the decision to start a low-FODMAP plan, I think it's important that you know about the other diets people try in order to combat digestive problems. Some are well researched and rooted in strong science, while others—well, let's just say the facts are a bit more questionable. But all of these diets have believers who, with an almost religious fervor, say that the plan they went on changed their life and turned their health around.

The next sections will outline each of the plans that you're most likely to hear about—what the diet consists of, who it might help, and the research behind it. I give you this for two reasons. First, whatever you decide, I want you to be as well informed as possible. Going low FODMAP can bring fantastic results for many with digestive problems. But maybe there's another plan that meets your needs better, depending on the details of your condition. So you should know what's out there before you commit. The second reason I want you to know about the other diets people go on to manage gut symptoms is that inevitably these plans will come up in conversation. Your best friend's sister's roommate is gluten-free, and she's 100 percent better—so "why not just go gluten-free?" Big Sister implores. Or the waitress at your favorite pizza place is eating only foods that are right for her blood type and thinks you should give it a try, too, and tries to convince you that it's really OK for you to keep those onions on your salad. Being aware of all of your options will allow you to calmly and rationally discuss the topic with other people (and defend yourself if need be) and help you solidify and own your dietary decision.

Here's the lowdown on some of the most common diets people try in the name of digestive wellness.

## Gluten-Free

A gluten-free diet eliminates gluten, a protein found in grains such as wheat, barley, and rye. Going gluten-free is the main treatment for celiac disease, an autoimmune disease in which eating gluten causes the body to attack itself, resulting in damage to the small intestine. There is also a lot of talk about a condition known as *nonceliac gluten sensitivity* (NCGS), also referred to as *wheat* or *gluten intolerance*, in which people have symptoms similar to those of a person with celiac disease but don't test positive for the condition; however, they notice an improvement when they eliminate gluten from their diets. NCGS is mysterious because there's a long list of symptoms a person might believe to be due to gluten—from bloating to diarrhea to migraines to tiredness—and there's currently no reliable test for it. The third category of people who may go gluten-free are those who have no known medical concern but believe that a gluten-free diet is healthier than a wheat-containing one. With all of the nutritious-looking gluten-free products available in stores and restaurants, it's easy to see how a person could come to believe that.

So who really belongs on a gluten-free diet? Gluten-free diets are no doubt necessary for a person with celiac disease, though it's possible that there is more going on in the gut, and that they might benefit from an additional diet tweak like low-FODMAP or the specific carbohydrate diet (discussed in a minute). The plot thickens for those with NCGS, as a 2013 study published in the journal *Gastroenterology* found that only 8 percent of the thirty-seven subjects who believed they were gluten intolerant felt a change in symptoms after altering the amount of gluten in their diet, while everyone in the study felt better from going low FODMAP. A newer study in the journal *Gut* uncovered that people with NCGS seem to have a leaky intestinal wall that allows food particles and bacteria to pass through, setting off an immune response in the body—so there is a biological explanation for this condition. While experts say that nonceliac gluten sensitivity or wheat intolerance likely does exist in 1 percent of the population, they haven't agreed on how to identify those people, and it seems many such people may benefit from going low FODMAP.

As for people with no health problems who think that going gluten-free is somehow healthier? That's unlikely to be the case. There's nothing inherently wrong with gluten, say experts, unless you're sensitive to it. What's more, gluten-free packaged foods like breads, crackers, and tortillas are often made with refined ingredients like white rice flour and can actually be less nutritious than their gluten-containing counterparts. So unless you actually need to be on a gluten-free diet, and depending on how you go about following it (are you eating kale salads and salmon or gluten-free muffins and cookies?), you may actually be doing your body a disservice.

*Bottom line:* Gluten-free diets are a must for anyone with celiac disease, though you might want to take it a step further and try low FODMAPs on top of gluten-free if you're still experiencing symptoms. Definitely talk with a registered dietitian nutritionist first to make sure you're not missing any hidden gluten sources. If you have ruled out celiac but believe your symptoms are due to gluten, it may be worth a try, but you may also want to see how you fare on a low-FODMAP plan.

## Grain-Free

A grain-free diet is one that goes beyond gluten-free, removing all grains and often pseudograins (seeds that are a lot like grains), including wheat, barley, corn, millet, oats, rice, sorghum, teff, triticale, amaranth, buckwheat, and quinoa. There isn't much research specifically on grain-free diets; however, researchers have looked a bit at the Paleo diet (see the next section), which is, by definition, a grain-free diet (it includes several other restrictions as well). Proponents of grain-free diets say they're beneficial for those with autoimmune issues and can help cut back on inflammation in the body. Other experts say it's refined grains that seem to have an inflammatory effect on the body, while whole grains may be different. Read on for more details.

*Bottom line:* It's possible that it could help if it cuts inflammation or eliminates your digestive triggers.

## Paleo Diet

Short for the Paleolithic diet, the Paleo diet—also known as the primal or ancestral diet—is based on the foods we humans supposedly ate back when we were cavemen and cavewomen: grass-fed meat; fish; seafood; fruits; vegetables; eggs; nuts; seeds; and oils from foods like olives, walnuts, flaxseeds, and coconuts. What you don't eat on a Paleo diet are any grains, legumes (beans, peas, peanuts), dairy foods (yogurt, cheese), potatoes, or refined sugar. While some devotees say that a Paleo diet has helped them get their IBS or IBD under control, I was unable to find any research supporting these claims. I did, however, find research that said it may help people with diabetes control their blood sugar, and that people on a Paleo diet seem to feel more satisfied by their meals.

*Bottom line:* A Paleo diet may eliminate your digestive triggers, and as a result you may feel better, but because you remove so many things all at once without reintroducing any, you won't know what the culprit is. Eating this way may, however, nudge you to eat fewer processed and more whole foods, which is a good thing, generally speaking.

## Autoimmune Paleo

Also known as the AIP protocol,

autoimmune Paleo is like a Paleo diet that just had a triple shot of espresso. In addition to the normal Paleo restrictions, AIP goes a step further and also cuts out eggs, nuts, seeds, nightshades (like eggplant), alcohol, and artificial sweeteners. Supporters say these foods are bad news for people with autoimmune diseases like celiac disease and rheumatoid arthritis, leading to leaky gut, inflammation, and sensitivity. A great source for learning more about the impact Paleo-inspired diets can have on autoimmune disease is Terry Wahls, a doctor who reversed symptoms of multiple sclerosis in large part through a Paleo-inspired plan.

*Bottom line:* If your gut problems are autoimmune-related (Crohn's disease, ulcerative colitis, celiac disease), it may be worth exploring this type of plan; a registered dietitian nutritionist who is well versed in elimination diets may be able to help you test out some principles of the AIP without pushing you off into the deep end or making you navigate a full-on, headfirst dive.

## Specific Carbohydrate Diet (SCD)

The specific carbohydrate diet (SCD) is intended for people with Crohn's disease, ulcerative colitis, celiac disease, diverticulitis, cystic fibrosis, and chronic diarrhea. While up until recently the research on the SCD was limited, evidence supporting its use has been growing. A study in the *Journal of the Academy of Nutrition and Dietetics* found that people with ulcerative colitis, indeterminate colitis (meaning it's not clear if the inflammation is due to Crohn's or ulcerative colitis), or Crohn's disease who chose to follow the specific carbohydrate diet said it was on average 91.3 percent effective at controlling acute flare symptoms and 92.1 percent effective at helping them maintain remission. Another small study on kids ages six to sixteen years old linked following the SCD with improvements in blood markers of inflammation as well as weight and height gains.

The catch: It's extremely restrictive. People on the SCD are allowed to eat only monosaccharide carbohydrates, or those made of one molecule, which are easily absorbed by the intestinal wall (the SCD diet is also gluten-free, which is why it's suitable for people with celiac disease). The theory behind it, similar to that of low FODMAPs, is that it limits carbohydrates whose breakdown products can serve as food for harmful bacteria, essentially starving the bacteria and rebalancing the gut as a result (the two diets take different approaches, however, and you'll find many contradictions between them).

The plan has a two- to five-day introductory phase in which you're encouraged to eat homemade chicken soup along with a very short list of approved foods like eggs, broiled fish, homemade gelatin, and dry-curd cottage cheese. After the first few days, you introduce more foods, carefully moving to a more liberal "legal/illegal" system where foods like ripe bananas with black spots and butternut squash are allowed, but canned pumpkin and potatoes are not. Also encouraged is a homemade yogurt that's fermented long enough to remove most of the lactose. Similar to low FODMAPs, it's tough to know off the top of your head what would work and what wouldn't work on the plan, so you'll have to consult the SCD bible, *Breaking the Vicious Cycle* by Elaine Gottschall, breakingtheviciouscycle.info, or the multitude of SCD diet blogs that have popped up.

*Bottom line:* May be worth a try if you have Crohn's disease or ulcerative colitis; if you decide to try it, know that the diet is incredibly restrictive—but the people it's worked for say it's well worth it. Meeting with a registered dietitian

nutritionist who is well versed in the SCD diet to help guide your choices is advised.

## GAPS Protocol

The protocol for GAPS, which stands for gut and psychology syndrome, grew out of the SCD diet and is centered around the belief that compromised gut health is the root cause of issues in the brain. Proponents of this very restrictive diet recommend it for people with learning disabilities and/or psychiatric and psychological disorders. GAPS is not, at the moment, backed by solid scientific research.

*Bottom line:* Some say it's worth considering if your gut issues overlap with brain or mental health issues. Work with a diet pro to determine what is right for you and to navigate this or any plan you choose.

## Low-Residue/Low-Fiber Diet

The low-residue/low-fiber diet limits the amount of fiber you're eating to no more than 10 to 15 grams per day in an effort to rein in bowel movements. *Low residue* is actually an outdated term (low fiber is more accurate), but you still may hear it being used. It may be prescribed to you if you have ulcerative colitis, Crohn's disease, diverticulitis, or other bowel inflammatory conditions; it's also used after intestinal surgeries. In addition to minimizing fiber-rich grains (like whole wheat bread, brown rice, and bran cereal), you also have to be mindful of the produce you're eating by choosing certain fruits and vegetables only if they're well cooked and avoiding others altogether. Other restrictions may include nuts, beans, and tough meats.

*Bottom line:* Before a procedure or after a surgery, this may be your best bet—take your doctor's advice. However, for long-term maintenance of your condition, there's a range of other diets that might help you manage symptoms while still allowing you to eat a more balanced diet.

## Blood-Type Diet

Popularized by a naturopathic doctor with a best-selling book, the blood-type plan is based on the theory that our bodies react differently to food depending on our blood types (A, B, O, and AB). Fans say that eating the foods that complement your blood can help you stay healthy and manage diseases, including gut disorders, and the topic of following a blood-type-influenced diet seems to come up a lot on IBS/IBD message boards. While the concept is totally intriguing, and there are people out there who feel it's worked for them, the research says otherwise: A review of sixteen blood-type diet studies published in the *American Journal of Clinical Nutrition* found that there is no evidence to support their claims.

*Bottom line:* There are far more well-researched options out there; stay tuned to see if the science evolves at all on this one.

# CHAPTER 4

# The LOW-FODMAP Plan:

## THE FOOD

If you have IBS or its symptoms, the reasons to try a low-FODMAP diet are solid:

**1.** For the majority of people with IBS, it works.

**2.** There are no side effects like you might experience from medication.

**3.** It doesn't cost you any money, aside from the normal expenses associated with food.

There is one drawback, however, and that's that a low-FODMAP plan takes some work. Knowing which foods are high in FODMAPs just by looking at them is virtually impossible, and once you do know which foods you can eat, you'll find that a low-FODMAP diet can be rather limiting.

That's where this section of the book comes in. I'm going to walk you through which foods you can and can't eat. I'll also make it easy for you to find meals and snacks that limit your intake of FODMAPs yet still give you plenty of options to keep your diet interesting—whether you're at a school cafeteria, in a restaurant, or in a dorm room. And I'll clue you in on some sneaky sources of FODMAPs so you won't get tripped up.

Another important detail about the low-FODMAP diet (one that many people miss!) is that the goal is not for you to stay on it for the rest of your life. Your mission, rather, is to eliminate high-FODMAP foods for long enough to feel an improvement in symptoms—two to six weeks—and then figure out precisely what's giving you a problem. With a little careful experimentation, which I'll help walk you through (see page 85), you can get to the bottom of what you can tolerate, and chances are, you'll be able to add back in some foods that are higher in FODMAPs as long as you keep the serving sizes small. Get this—an overly restrictive diet may actually be *bad* for gut health in the long run—even if it's helping you feel better right now. So I'm going to help you experiment in a careful and measured way so you can arrive at a less-fussy diet that you can live with in the long term.

## GET TO KNOW THE SYSTEM: GO, SLOW, AND NO

I admit, this is all a lot to digest (pardon the pun). So to make it a little bit easier to swallow (OK, OK!) I've broken things down into three categories: Go, Slow, and No.

- *Go* foods are foods that contain few or no FODMAPs and aren't likely to affect your digestive symptoms—think of them as green-light foods that you can continue eating normal-size portions of without much concern.

- *Slow* foods may contain a limited amount of FODMAPs but shouldn't cause a problem *as long as you are careful to eat them in moderation.* Portion size is key with these foods, and we'll tell you what a portion should look like so you can eat them and avoid any nasty side effects. These are your yellow-light foods—you can eat them, but you have to slow down a bit and exercise caution. Also included in the slow section are foods that aren't high in FODMAPs but may cause digestive distress for other reasons, so you should proceed carefully.

- *No* foods are the ones that are loaded with FODMAPs. At the start, you'll want to avoid them completely—think of them as red-light foods. The good news: After two to six weeks of staying away from these foods, we'll carefully reintroduce them to determine what you can and can't tolerate.

## Size Matters

Just because a food is considered low in FODMAPs doesn't necessarily mean you can eat a supersized portion. There are some foods that do have FODMAPs in them, but a reasonably sized portion will keep the offending carbs to enough of a minimum that they shouldn't negatively affect you. Take a food like avocado. One half of an avocado has high amounts of the polyol sorbitol and is considered a high-FODMAP food. Cut that half avocado into quarters, though, and you can comfortably eat that eighth of an avocado. In food terms, that means a chips-and-guac appetizer is a no-no. But a little bit of mashed avocado on your turkey sandwich with gluten-free bread (if you measure it carefully)? Absolutely!

For the first few weeks of your low-FODMAP diet, eating Go and Slow foods only is important because it will give you the opportunity to find out what will work for you. This commitment will help get your gut back on track and find some—if not total—relief from your symptoms before you start adding No foods back in. Remember: *The end goal is not for you to be on a low-FODMAP diet for life, but rather to pinpoint the foods that give you trouble and learn to eat those in amounts that your body can handle.* But that's later. For now, we're going to Go Low. Let's go!

## A Go Low Must-Have

The first thing I want you to do as you begin to Go Low if you have a smartphone is to download the Monash University Low FODMAP Diet app (for more on the app, see page 189). Even though it's on the expensive side for an app ($7.99 when this book went to press), once you have it you can look up any food that crosses your path and the experts at Monash University will tell you whether the food is low, moderate, or high in FODMAPs. It will also tell you the approved serving sizes. Because the lab where the food is being tested is in Australia, the database is heavily weighted toward Aussie foods (and you may have to Google some Australian food names—who knew that they call bell peppers *capsicum*?!), however the team in Melbourne is working to expand its international offerings. But even without being able to know for sure if your favorite brand of gluten-free cookies from Trader Joe's is safe, the app is still incredibly valuable for anyone following a low-FODMAP plan.

I've included a list of Go Low–approved foods on pages 55 to 58, a list of No foods that you'll need to skip while in phase one (pages 60 to 61), a grocery list of approved foods (pages 62 to 65), and more than thirty Go Low recipes in Chapter 9. But no matter how much information I provide you with, it's impossible to give you a comprehensive list of low-FODMAP foods and corresponding serving sizes. The reason? Researchers are constantly testing and measuring foods to find out their FODMAP status. The most thorough and up-to-date source for that is the Monash University Low FODMAP Diet app, and that's why I urge you or someone in your family to get it to use as a reference. If there's anything you're not sure about, consult the frequently updated and very comprehensive app before eating.

## Go Foods

Because the list of foods you can't eat on a low-FODMAP diet can feel overwhelming, let's begin with the foods you *can* eat. As of this printing, here are the Go foods to focus on eating more of during phase one of your low-FODMAP diet. I've included the serving size recommended by the experts at Monash—for the most part, this is the amount you should stick with per meal or snack. However, a U in brackets—[U] (for unlimited!)—appears next to the foods that the experts say you can eat as much as you'd like of (don't go too crazy on alfalfa sprouts, now!):

### VEGETABLES

| FOOD | SERVING SIZE |
|---|---|
| Alfalfa sprouts [U] | ½ cup (15 g) |
| Arugula | 1 cup (35 g) |
| Bell pepper | ½ cup (50 g) sliced |
| Bok choy | 1 cup (85 g) chopped |
| Broccoli | ½ cup (45 g) florets |
| Cabbage, common—green or red | 1 cup (95 g) chopped |
| Carrot [U] | 1 medium |
| Celery root | ½ celery root |
| Chard [U] | 1 cup (115 g) chopped |
| Chives | 1 tablespoon chopped |
| Cucumber | ½ cup (65 g) chopped |
| Eggplant | ½ cup (40 g) chopped |
| Fennel | ½ cup (50 g) chopped |
| Ginger root | 1 teaspoon grated |
| Green beans | 12 green beans |
| Kale, cooked [U] | 1 cup (135 g) chopped |
| Lettuce, butter or red | 1 cup (35 g) chopped |
| Lettuce, iceberg | 1 cup (70 g) chopped |
| Okra | 6 pods |
| Olives, black or green | 15 small |

*chart continues . . .*

| | |
|---|---|
| Parsnip [U] | ½ cup (60 g) sliced |
| Potato | 1 medium |
| Radish | 2 radishes |
| Scallions (green onions) green tops only | 1 bunch |
| Spaghetti squash [U] | 1 cup (155 g) cooked strands |
| Spinach, baby | 1 cup (35 g) |
| Squash, yellow | 2 squashes |
| Tomato, cherry or grape | 4 tomatoes |
| Tomato, common or plum | 1 small |
| Turnip | 1 cup (65 g) chopped |
| Water chestnuts | ½ cup (55 g) sliced |
| Zucchini | ½ cup (65 g) chopped |

## FRUITS

| FOOD | SERVING SIZE |
|---|---|
| Banana, ripe or firm | 1 medium |
| Blueberries | 20 berries |
| Cantaloupe | ½ cup (90 g) chopped |
| Carambola (star fruit) | 1 medium |
| Clementine | 1 medium |
| Grapes, red or green | 1 cup (150 g) |
| Guava, ripe | 1 medium |
| Honeydew melon | ½ cup (90 g) chopped |
| Kiwifruit, green or gold, peeled | 2 small |
| Lemon | 1 teaspoon of juice |
| Lime | 1 teaspoon of juice |
| Mandarin orange | 2 small |
| Orange | 1 medium |
| Passionfruit | pulp of 1 passionfruit |
| Pineapple | 1 cup (140 g) chopped |
| Raspberry | 10 berries |
| Rhubarb | 1 cup (130 g) chopped |
| Strawberry | 10 strawberries |

## DAIRY/DAIRY ALTERNATIVE

| FOOD | SERVING SIZE |
|---|---|
| Cheese, Brie | 2 wedges (1.4 ounces/40 g total) |
| Cheese, Camembert | 2 wedges (1.4 ounces/40 g total) |
| Cheese, cheddar | 2 slices (1.4 ounces/40 g total) |
| Cheese, Colby | 2 slices (1.4 ounces/40 g total) |
| Cheese, cottage | ¼ cup (35 g) |
| Cheese, feta | ½ cup (125 g) crumbled |
| Cheese, goat | ½ cup (60 g) crumbled |
| Cheese, Havarti | 2 slices (1.9 ounces/54 g total) |
| Cheese, mozzarella | ½ cup (60 g) grated |
| Cheese, Parmesan | ½ cup (60 g) grated |
| Cheese, Romano | ½ cup (60 g) grated |
| Cheese, Swiss | 2 slices (1.9 ounces/54 g total) |
| Cream, whipped | ½ cup (60 g) |
| Milk, almond | 1 cup (240 ml) |
| Milk, coconut (canned) | ½ cup (120 ml) |
| Milk, hemp | 1 cup (240 ml) |
| Milk, lactose-free | 1 cup (240 ml) |
| Milk, rice | ¾ cup (180 ml) |
| Yogurt, goat's milk | 6 ounces (170 g) |
| Yogurt, lactose-free | 6 ounces (170 g) |

## PROTEIN [U]*

| FOOD | SERVING SIZE |
|------|--------------|
| Beef, cooked | 4.4 ounces (125 g) |
| Chicken, cooked | 4.4 ounces (125 g) |
| Turkey, cooked | 4.4 ounces (125 g) |
| Eggs | 2 medium |
| Fish, any type (canned) | 3.7 ounces (105 g) |
| Fish, any type (fresh) | 3.5 ounces (100 g) cooked, 4 ounces (115 g) raw |
| Lamb, cooked | 4.4 ounces (125 g) |
| Lentils (canned) | ½ cup (45 g) |
| Pork, cooked | 4.4 ounces (125 g) |
| Shrimp | 10 small (2 ounces/60 g total) |
| Tofu, firm | $^2/_3$ cup (160 g) cubed |
| Tempeh | 3.5 ounces (100 g) |

*Because strictly protein foods (read: meat from any animal, including fish and shellfish, and eggs) don't contain any carbohydrates, you likely can eat as much as you'd like of any type without consequence—including those not listed above, like bacon, crab, mussels, and oysters—even though they haven't all been tested separately for their FODMAP content. Just beware of protein foods that are cooked with high-FODMAP foods (like a garlic marinade) or combined with them (like onions in sausages or hot dogs).

## CARBOHYDRATES*

| FOOD | SERVING SIZE |
|------|--------------|
| Bread, gluten-free | 2 slices |
| Bread, sourdough** | 2 slices |
| Buckwheat groats | ¾ cup (135 g) cooked |
| Corn chips, plain | 1.5 ounces (50 g) |
| Cornflakes, gluten-free | 1 cup (35 g) |
| Pasta, gluten-free | 1 cup (145 g) cooked |
| Polenta (cornmeal) | 1 cup (255 g) cooked |
| Popcorn, plain | 3½ cups (60 g) popped |
| Rice, brown or white | 1 cup (180 g) cooked |
| Rice cakes | 2 cakes |
| Rice noodles | 1 cup (220 g) cooked |
| Tortilla chips | About 25 (50 g) |
| Tortillas, corn | 2 small |
| Quinoa | 1 cup (155 g) cooked |
| Quinoa flakes hot cereal | 1 cup (50 g) uncooked |

*Check ingredients lists to ensure that all ingredients used are Go Low approved.

**Not just any sourdough will cut it, though. For more details on how to choose the right sourdough, see page 136.

## NUTS AND SEEDS

| FOOD | SERVING SIZE |
| --- | --- |
| Chia seeds | 2 tablespoons |
| Macadamia nuts | 20 nuts |
| Peanut butter* | 2 tablespoons |
| Peanuts | 32 nuts |
| Pine nuts | 1 tablespoon |
| Pumpkin seeds | 2 tablespoons |
| Sesame seeds | 1 tablespoon |

*Always stick with peanut butter that has no more than two ingredients: peanuts and salt. Some companies add unexpected ingredients that (a) you just don't need and (b) might mess with your stomach.

## FATS AND OILS*

| FOOD | SERVING SIZE |
| --- | --- |
| Butter | 1 tablespoon |
| Margarine | 1 tablespoon |
| Mayonnaise | 2 tablespoons |
| Oil, avocado | 1 tablespoon |
| Oil, canola | 1 tablespoon |
| Oil, coconut | 1 tablespoon |
| Oil, olive | 1 tablespoon |
| Oil, peanut | 1 tablespoon |
| Oil, sesame | 1 tablespoon |
| Oil, sunflower | 1 tablespoon |
| Oil, vegetable | 1 tablespoon |

*Pure fats and oils by nature don't contain any FODMAPs. However, too much fat can mess with your digestion, so you can't use them to excess. Be mindful of how much you're eating.

## CONDIMENTS*

| FOOD | SERVING SIZE |
| --- | --- |
| Apple cider vinegar | 2 tablespoons |
| Asafetida powder | ¼ teaspoon |
| Barbecue sauce | 2 tablespoons |
| Capers | 1 tablespoon |
| Fish sauce | 1 tablespoon |
| Herbs, dried | ¼ cup (5 g) |
| Herbs, fresh | 1 cup (15 g) |
| Maple syrup | 2 tablespoons |
| Miso paste | 2 teaspoons |
| Mustard | 1 tablespoon |
| Oyster sauce | 1 tablespoon |
| Rice wine vinegar | 2 tablespoons |
| Soy sauce | 2 tablespoons |
| Spices | 1 teaspoon ground |
| Worcestershire sauce | 2 tablespoons |

*Read labels to make sure condiments don't include any of the No ingredients listed on pages 60 to 61. Note that onion and garlic powders are not permitted when you're going low, so look out for them in herb and spice blends as well as in barbecue sauce.

# Slow Foods

You are permitted to eat the following foods during phase one, as long as you take extra precaution to keep their serving sizes to a minimum.

## PROTEIN

| FOOD | SERVING SIZE |
| --- | --- |
| Chickpeas (canned) | ¼ cup (40 g) |
| Lentils, boiled | ¼ cup (25 g) |
| Lentils (canned) | ½ cup (45 g) |

## VEGETABLES

| FOOD | SERVING SIZE |
| --- | --- |
| Artichoke hearts (canned) | 2 tablespoons |
| Avocado | $1/8$ avocado or less |
| Brussels sprouts | 2 sprouts |
| Butternut squash | ¼ cup (30 g) chopped |
| Celery | ¼ medium stalk |
| Endive | 4 leaves |
| Pumpkin, canned | ¼ cup (60 g) |
| Tomatoes, sun-dried | 2 pieces |

## CARBOHYDRATES

| FOOD | SERVING SIZE |
| --- | --- |
| Potato chips, plain | 1 ounce (30 g) |
| Pretzels, gluten-free | ½ cup (20 g) |
| Puffed amaranth cereal | ¼ cup (10 g) |
| Puffed rice cereal | ½ cup (15 g) |
| Quick oats | ¼ cup (25 g) |

## FRUITS

| FOOD | SERVING SIZE |
| --- | --- |
| Coconut, dried | ¼ cup (20 g) |
| Coconut, fresh | ½ cup (50 g) |
| Cranberries, dried | 1 tablespoon |

## NUTS/SEEDS

| FOOD | SERVING SIZE |
| --- | --- |
| Brazil nuts | 10 nuts |
| Hazelnuts | 10 nuts |
| Pecans | 10 halves |
| Sunflower seeds | 2 teaspoons (shelled) |
| Walnuts | 10 halves |

## DAIRY/DAIRY ALTERNATIVES

| FOOD | SERVING SIZE |
| --- | --- |
| Cheese, American | 1 slice |
| Cheese, ricotta | 2 tablespoons |
| Cream | ½ cup (120 ml) |

## CONDIMENTS

| FOOD | SERVING SIZE |
| --- | --- |
| Balsamic vinegar | 1 tablespoon |

The information in these charts was adapted from the Monash University Low FODMAP Diet app and up to date as of this book's publication.

## Gluten-Free Does Not Equal Low FODMAP

Gluten is a protein found in wheat, barley, and rye. People on a low-FODMAP plan cannot eat wheat because it has a high level of oligosaccharides (the *O* in *FOD-MAP*). Because gluten-free products by nature don't include any wheat, when you find them on the shelf, there's a chance that they're safe for someone who is Going Low. However, it's not a guarantee. The reason? Many gluten-free ingredients are not low FODMAP. Take Banza, a delicious gluten-free pasta that is made from chickpea flour. Chickpeas are also high in oligosaccharides, so sadly, you can tell right away that Banza isn't low FODMAP. Other gluten-free food products like the breads from Rudi's Gluten-Free Bakery may seem OK at first—until you realize that they are sweetened with honey (some also include inulin, another no-no). Bottom line: Use gluten-free labels to narrow down what foods might work for you; then scour the ingredients lists to get the final word.

Some foods are not necessarily high in FODMAPs; however, they can affect people with sensitive guts. Proceed with caution in particular when eating or drinking tea, coffee, chocolate/cocoa, carbonated beverages such as seltzer, oils, fried foods, and alcohol.

## No Foods

You'll skip the foods in these lists during the first two to six weeks of Going Low. Don't worry—you'll be able to reintroduce some of them after that, so they may not be out of your life for good.

Vegetables: artichoke leaves, asparagus, beets, cauliflower, corn, garlic, leeks, mushrooms, onions, savoy cabbage, scallions (white parts), shallots, snap peas, snow peas, soybeans, taro

Fruit: apples, apricots, Asian pears, blackberries, boysenberries, cherries, currants, dates, figs, grapefruit, unripe guava, lychees, mangos, nectarines, peaches, pears, persimmons, plums, pomegranates, watermelon; dried fruit (with the exception of small amounts of dried cranberries and coconut)

Dairy/dairy alternatives: buttermilk, cream cheese, kefir, milk, oat milk, sour cream, soy milk, yogurt (cow's milk or soy)

Protein: anything breaded or seasoned with garlic or onion; beans like kidney, black, and butter (exceptions: canned chickpeas or lentils, and cooked dried lentils in small amounts); falafel; lima beans; mung beans; silken tofu; soybeans

Carbohydrates: amaranth, barley, bread, bulgur, couscous, cornflakes cereal (regular), freekeh, granola, pasta (regular), crispy rice cereal, rye, spelt, wheat bran, wheat flour. (Note: Many grain products that are typically high-FODMAP have gluten-free equivalents that are Go foods; check the ingredients on the label to be certain.)

Nuts and seeds: Almonds, cashews, pistachios

Condiments/extras: Agave, carob, chamomile tea, cream sauce, garlic powder, garlic salt, honey, hummus, jam, jelly, ketchup, onion powder, spice mixes and rubs (most contain onion or garlic), tahini, tomato paste, tomato sauce, tzatziki

Packaged-food ingredients: agave, chicory root, fruit juice (except pure cranberry juice, which is OK), FOS, garlic (including garlic powder and garlic salt), high-fructose corn syrup, honey, inulin, isomalt, mannitol, maltitol, milk, sorbitol, soy (whole soy— exceptions: firm tofu, soy sauce), onion (including onion powder and onion salt), xylitol

# GO LOW, GO SHOPPING!

Making this program easy for you to follow is my main goal. That's why I put together this list for you (or your parent) to reference when you go to the grocery store. It's divided up by category of food so you can find things easily. Keep in mind that most packaged foods in the United States haven't been tested for FODMAPs, but these are products that I and other low-FODMAP enthusiasts have scoured to make sure they use only Go Low ingredients, which means they shouldn't pose a problem for you. If you're not feeling great after eating any, however, you may want to dial back the packaged foods and stick with simple one-ingredient foods that have been tested for their FODMAP content.

## Grains and Cereals

### FOODS

- Corn tortillas (make sure they don't contain wheat flour)
- Gluten-free pasta (I love the quinoa/ brown rice ones at Trader Joe's; other good options are the brown rice ones made by Tinkyada and Jovial)
- Potato chips
- Popcorn kernels (see Olive Oil and Herb Stovetop Popcorn, page 186)
- Rice (brown or white)
- Rice noodles
- Tortilla chips
- Quinoa

### BRAND-NAME PRODUCTS

- 88 Acres seed bars (Triple Berry* or Chocolate & Sea Salt)
- Ancient Harvest Traditional Polenta (precooked in the shape of a log; look for the plain flavor, as some others contain garlic)
- Be Nice low-FODMAP bars (available online)
- Bob's Red Mill Rolled Oats
- Boomchickapop Sea Salt Popcorn
- Cheerios
- Erewhon brown rice cereal
- Erewhon Crispy Corn Flakes Cereal
- EnviroKidz Gorilla Munch Cereal
- EnviroKidz Peanut Butter Panda Puffs Cereal

*Triple Berry does contain No food currants, but in amounts small enough for most low FODMAPers to tolerate.

TRY THIS

## The Great Garlic Workaround

Fructans, the tummy-twisting oligosaccharides in onions and garlic, are water soluble; in other words, water pulls them out from the vegetable's fiber. When exposed to oil, however, the fructans do the opposite—they stay put. So while you can't eat pieces of garlic or onion when you Go Low, and you can't simply pull the translucent strands out of your French onion soup because the fructans are already in the broth, here's what you can do to add fructan-free flavor to your dishes if you really miss that garlic or onion taste: Sauté a clove of garlic or big pieces of onion in oil, then remove them before you add the rest of the ingredients to the oil.

- Glutino gluten-free pretzels
- Lundberg brown rice cakes
- Nature's Path original Hot Oatmeal packets
- Nature Valley crunchy peanut butter/cinnamon granola bars
- Popchips (sea salt flavor, 1 ounce/30 g)
- Qi'a Superfoods Superseeds & Grains Hot Oatmeal
- Quaker Oats plain instant oatmeal packets
- Quinn microwave popcorn
- Real Foods Corn Thins
- Snyder's of Hanover gluten-free pretzels
- Suzie's Thin Cakes, lightly salted corn
- Udi's gluten-free white sandwich bread
- Udi's gluten-free frozen pizza crust

## Dairy and Dairy Alternatives
- Lactose-free yogurt
- Lactose-free kefir
- Lactose-free cream cheese
- Lactose-free cheese
- Lactose-free milk
- Unsweetened almond milk

## Protein
All meats and fish, as long as they aren't marinated or combined in any way with high-FODMAP foods like garlic and onions (including garlic and onion powders)

### Can I Use Artificial Sweeteners on a Low-FODMAP Plan?

Erythritol, the sweet substance used in those little green Truvia packets alongside stevia leaf extract, appears to be pretty benign as far as your gut is concerned—on its own, that is. When consumed alongside the fruit sugar fructose (like in a blended smoothie or sprinkled on a grapefruit half), however, the sweetener increases fructose malabsorption, according to research from Louisiana Tech University. What's more, other research has found that various artificial sweeteners may alter gut bacteria in a way that affects metabolism—and not for the better. Bottom line: Artificial sweeteners may be affecting you in ways you'd never realize. What's more, you don't really need them since you're OK to use sweeteners like sugar and maple syrup in moderation. I suggest you skip artificial sweeteners when you Go Low and beyond.

# Go Low Snacks

If you're used to snacking on bagel chips and hummus or Pop-Tarts, getting started on a low-FODMAP plan can feel overwhelming. But there are plenty of delish munchies you can have instead that will be much easier on your belly. Why not try some of these:

- 88 Acres seed bars (Triple Berry or Chocolate & Sea Salt)
- Go Low–approved gluten-free pretzels (like Snyder's of Hanover or Glutino)
- Potato chips (plain salted ones are OK, like Kettle Brand sea salt; stay away from flavored ones)
- Sea salt Popchips (1 ounce/30 g)
- Popcorn
- Rice cake with peanut butter and banana
- Rice crackers and low-lactose cheese
- ProNourish Low FODMAP Nutritional Drink
- No-Bake Peanut Butter Bars (page 154)
- Peanut Butter–Chocolate Power Balls (page 181)
- Chocolate-Covered Strawberry Shake (page 183)
- Lactose-free yogurt with low-FODMAP berries

**OTHER FOODS YOU MAY WANT TO PICK UP:**

- Firm or extra firm tofu
- Eggs
- Nuts: macadamia nuts, peanuts/peanut butter (like Smucker's Natural), pecans, walnuts
- Seeds: chia, hemp, pumpkin, sunflower

## Produce

- Arugula
- Bananas
- Bell peppers
- Blueberries
- Bok choy
- Cabbage, green or red
- Carrots
- Cucumbers
- Eggplant
- Fennel
- Grapes
- Green beans
- Kale
- Lemons

- Lettuce
- Oranges
- Parsnips
- Potatoes
- Raspberries
- Scallions (use green parts only)
- Squash, yellow
- Strawberries
- Tomatoes
- Zucchini

## Other

- Rao's Sensitive Formula Marinara Sauce or FODY Low FODMAP Marinara Sauce
- Soy sauce or tamari, which is similar to soy sauce (look for gluten-free, if you are sensitive)
- Individual packets of San J gluten-free tamari (if you are gluten-free)
- Nori (seaweed) sheets
- Maple syrup
- Gluten-free baking mix like Bob's Red Mill 1-to-1 or King Arthur Flour Gluten-Free All-Purpose Baking Mix (make sure all ingredients are Go Low–approved; some mixes—including Bob's Red Mill's gluten-free all-purpose baking flour, a different blend from the 1-to-1—contain red-light ingredients like garbanzo bean flour).

## GREAT MEAL OPTIONS ON THE LOW-FODMAP PLAN

Chances are, you'll be able to add a range of Slow foods back in without symptoms. But until then, my job is to make phase one—the elimination phase—as easy for you as possible. Now, you may not be used to taking the lead in meal preparation (or keeping a close watch on what's being served to you). If that's you, this can be even more annoying than the restrictions themselves! That's why I've included lots of recipes and ideas to make this new role super easy. To that end, here's an example of how you might eat for one week during Go Low phase one, or the elimination phase. Think on the bright side: Being more involved in food prep can help ensure you get to eat the foods you want to eat (within the parameters of Going Low, of course), and it will definitely help you stick with the plan and feel better. See Chapter 9 for more food ideas.

## GOING LOW ON THE GO

Bringing a meal with you is always a smart idea while you're Going Low. The reason: You know exactly what's in the food you're eating. Here are some easy-to-make meals you can throw together before you head out the door.

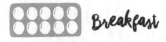 ## Breakfast

- 1 (6-ounce/170 g) container lactose-free vanilla yogurt topped with 20 (30 g) blueberries
- 2 Egg Flowers (page 148)
- Quinoa hot cereal (½ cup/25 g dried, prepared with water) topped with ½ banana, 2 tablespoons walnuts, and 1 teaspoon brown sugar
- 2 eggs scrambled with ½ cup (20 g) baby spinach and topped with

- 2 tablespoons shredded Parmesan + 1 slice gluten-free bread, toasted
- Banana-Blueberry Smoothie (page 147)
- 1 cup (50 g) gluten-free cereal with ⅓ cup (80 ml) lactose-free milk or unsweetened almond milk and 5 (70 g) medium sliced strawberries
- 2 slices gluten-free bread, toasted and topped with 2 tablespoons peanut butter and 2 strawberries, sliced thinly

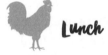 ## Lunch

- 2 slices gluten-free bread with 3 ounces (85 g) sliced turkey breast, 1 teaspoon mayonnaise, 2 pieces lettuce, and 1 tomato slice + 1 ounce (30 g) Popchips
- Cheddar quesadilla on a corn tortilla with ½ small tomato and 1 tablespoon chopped cilantro
- Salad with lettuce, cucumber, red bell pepper, and carrots, topped with

3 ounces (85 g) grilled chicken, ¼ cup (60 g) crumbled feta, 1 to 2 tablespoons olive oil and lemon juice dressing (see page 81 for how to make a Go Low–safe salad at any salad bar)
- Carrot and Coriander Soup (page 158)
- Mix-and-Match, a.k.a. the Bento (see page 68)
- Vietnamese Noodle Salad (page 160)
- Open-Face Egg Mash (page 161)

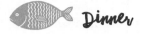 ## Dinner

- 1 cup (145 g) gluten-free pasta tossed with 2 tablespoons olive oil, 8 black olives, a handful of baby spinach, and 3 ounces (85 g) sliced grilled chicken
- 4-ounce (115 g) salmon fillet served with a lemon wedge + ½ cup (65 g) zucchini, sautéed and topped with a sprinkle of Parmesan + 1 medium potato (120 g), cubed and roasted
- 3 ounces (85 g) tofu stir-fried with 1 tablespoon soy sauce, 1 teaspoon sesame oil, and 1 cup (100 g) total chopped zucchini, red pepper, or yellow pepper + ½ cup (90 g) cooked brown rice
- Creamy (But Cream-Free) Tomato-Basil Soup (page 157) + a grilled cheese sandwich with lactose-free cheese and gluten-free bread
- Pesto Noodles and Zoodles (page 167)
- Mini Polenta Pizzas (page 172)
- Thai Quinoa Bowl (page 174)

 ## Snack

- 1 lactose-free cheese stick
- Chocolate-Covered Strawberry Shake (page 183)
- ½ banana rolled in 2 teaspoons sunflower seeds
- ½ cup (70 g) pineapple cubes tossed with cinnamon
- 1 hard-boiled egg
- ½ cup (75 g) frozen grapes
- ½ cup (20 g) gluten-free pretzels with 1 tablespoon peanut butter

## Sandwiches

Make all sandwiches on a Go Low–approved bread (like Udi's white sandwich)

- Peanut butter and banana
- Turkey breast and lettuce with up to 2 tablespoons mayo
- Ham and cheddar cheese
- Tuna with up to 2 tablespoons mayo

## Cold Salads

**Kale and Sunflower Salad:** 1 cup (15 g) chopped kale with olive oil and lemon juice (it sounds silly, but "massage" the kale until the leaves begin to wilt—it will help them become softer), tossed with 4 cherry tomatoes, quartered, and sprinkled with 2 teaspoons sunflower seeds and 2 tablespoons grated Parmesan

**Chicken Rice Bowl:** ¾ cup (135 g) cooked brown rice topped with ½ cup (15 g) chopped romaine lettuce, 2 tablespoons chopped cucumber, 2 tablespoons chopped carrots, 3 ounces (85 g) chopped grilled chicken breast, 2 teaspoons chopped walnuts, and olive oil and lemon juice

**Summer Pasta Salad:** 1 cup (145 g) cooked brown rice fusilli pasta (warm or cold) mixed with ½ cup (15 g) baby arugula, ¼ cup (60 g) crumbled feta, 4 cherry tomatoes, quartered, 10 small olives, halved, and a drizzle of olive oil

## Mix-and-Match, a.k.a. the Bento

This is my favorite option, mainly because it works even when I think I have no food in the house—in other words, often. A little of this, a little of that, and suddenly you have a well-balanced, satisfying meal. I call this "the bento" because it mimics the style of lunches popular in Japan, where people pack individual foods in boxes with multiple compartments (called bento boxes) to build a complete meal. Use the lists below to plan your meal—put the approved Go Low serving size of each component in a ziplock bag or use a cool bento box you can get from companies like Yumbox, Bentgo, and Laptop Lunches (search "bento" on Amazon and you'll find loads of options). Choose one food from each category, and you're good to go.

**Protein:** Hard-boiled egg, lactose-free yogurt, lactose-free cheese stick, peanut butter, cubed firm tofu, deli turkey, deli ham, deli roast beef

## Get Toasty

Gluten-free bread pretty much always tastes better in toast form. I'm not sure why, but I've yet to find a gluten-free bread where this isn't the case (if you find one, please let me know—I'd love to try it). I highly recommend toasting any gluten-free bread before you eat it or pack it for later.

**Grain:** Mary's Gone Crackers original rice crackers, rice cakes, brown rice, Food Should Taste Good Multigrain Tortilla Chips

**Vegetable:** Red, green, or yellow bell pepper; cucumber; carrots; fennel; zucchini; yellow (summer) squash

**Fruits:** Blueberries, cantaloupe, clementine, grapes, kiwi, honeydew, pineapple, raspberries, strawberries

# WAYS TO BOOST FLAVOR WHILE GOING LOW

Just because Going Low means eliminating flavorful ingredients like garlic and onions (for at least phase one), it doesn't mean living without food that does backflips on your taste buds. Here is a list of ingredients you can use to accessorize any meal and make it shine.

- Apple cider vinegar (2 tablespoons)
- Asafetida powder (¼ teaspoon; just make sure this Indian spice that people use to stand in for garlic/onion flavor isn't mixed with any other ingredients, as it sometimes is)
- Capers (1 tablespoon)
- Cocoa powder (2 teaspoons)
- Fish sauce (like Thai Kitchen brand, 1 tablespoon)
- Fresh or dried herbs: basil, cilantro, lemongrass, parsley, rosemary, tarragon, thyme
- Ginger root, minced (1 teaspoon)
- Lemon juice (1 teaspoon)
- Lime juice (1 teaspoon)
- Miso paste (2 teaspoons)
- Mustard (1 tablespoon)
- Oyster sauce (1 tablespoon)
- Rice wine vinegar (2 tablespoons)
- Spices, ground (1 teaspoon):

cardamom, chili powder, cinnamon, cloves, cumin, nutmeg, paprika, pepper, turmeric
- Soy sauce or tamari (2 tablespoons)
- Wasabi (1 teaspoon)
- Worcestershire sauce (2 tablespoons)

# GOING LOW AT RESTAURANTS AND THE DINING HALL

Americans on average dine out four to five times per week, according to a survey by Zagat (and that's not counting breakfast—what?!). Even if you eat at restaurants or fast-food places far less than that, chances are you'll have to eat out at some point during your time on the Go Low plan. No surprise, eating at restaurants can be tough while you're on a low-FODMAP plan, or any restricted diet for that matter. And while it won't always be possible, I do recommend avoiding eating out as much as you can during phase one of Going Low, because it can be so hard to control what you're eating at restaurants.

## Eating Out Survival Guide

So what's so hard about eating out? Depending on the cuisine, chefs may use garlic and onions to start many recipes, and you may never know if a sauce or soup is thickened with flour or made creamy with milk. And while more and more establishments offer gluten-free options, as you know, gluten-free does not equal low FODMAP (see page 60).

But you live in the real world, and eating out while you're challenging yourself to stick to a low-FODMAP plan may be impossible to avoid. Here are some strategies you can use to enjoy eating out while you Go Low.

*Be prepared:* Most restaurants have menus online. Take the time before you go to see what's on the menu and think out a game plan. Consider what items sound like they'd be safe, and make a mental note of what questions you'll need to ask the server, like "Does that salad have onions in it?" or "Can I get the chicken prepared without the sauce?" Going to a chain restaurant? There are some pros and cons. On the bright side, some companies actually list ingredients online so you'll know exactly what's in anything you might order. The negative of chain restaurants is that food is often prepared only a certain way, and there's not much room for the kitchen to whip up something special for you. Chances are, however,

## RESTAURANT REALITIES

"I remind myself that I'm there to spend time with friends or family, not to have a perfect meal."

"Sometimes it's challenging to find food at certain restaurants."

"It's hard to watch everyone eat foods that you love but can't have."

"I tell myself it's for the best that I eat this way, and that makes it much easier."

"It frustrates me when people assume I'm just on a fad diet. But I know it's how I need to eat."

with a little detective work you'll be able to find something—and if nothing else, you'll be prepared for whatever may be coming your way.

*Plain Jane your order:* It's kind of boring, sure. But it's safe. Try to stick with a meal where you can see all of the ingredients, like grilled chicken with wild rice and spinach, rather than a meal that's all cooked together like chicken and rice stew. Ask for your meals to be prepared as simply as possible, without seasonings. Mention explicitly that you can't eat garlic and onions, as they have a way of sneaking their way into food at restaurants.

*Always ask for "on the side":* Salad dressings and sauces can contain ingredients that won't work for you. Ask for your salad and other veggies "undressed," then add your own olive oil and lemon juice for flavor.

*Bring in some reinforcements:* Depending on where you're eating, different meal supplements can help round out your plate and turn your food in a feast. Sushi or Chinese restaurant? If you're gluten-free, packets of gluten-free soy sauce or tamari are crucial. A diner or deli? A bag of rice crackers can turn a plate of plain lunch meat and veggies into do-it-yourself mini sandwiches.

# Kidding Around

Children's menus often keep things far simpler and plainer than adult menus. Maybe it's been a couple of years since you've ordered from a kids' menu, but now's a good opportunity to embrace your inner child and go for the kiddie meal, if it provides you with more transparent options.

## Go-To Meals at Various Restaurants

Here are a few tips for what to eat at different types of restaurants while you Go Low.

Italian: Garlic and onions and dairy, oh my! Italian cuisine is one of my favorites, but it's a tough nut to crack when it comes to eating low FODMAPs. Looking through the menus of my favorite local Italian restaurants, however, I noticed some surprises. More and more restaurants are offering gluten-free pasta, which may be suitable for you (double-check to make sure it doesn't contain any chickpea flour or other FODMAP ingredients)—as long as the chef can prepare it with olive oil or butter sauce (remember, no garlic). Grilled chicken, sautéed shrimp, a side of broccoli (½ cup/45 g), and a few bites of sautéed spinach could all work well, as

long as the chef can meet your no-garlic request. And if he doesn't listen, you're not doomed—simply pick out the garlic pieces. As long as you don't eat the garlic flesh, you're OK. Pizza, sadly, is a no-go.

Japanese: A winner! Few restaurant meals leave less to the imagination than the Japanese specialty sushi, where you can see the ingredients laid out in front of you right on the menu: your favorite raw fish—yellowtail, salmon, tuna—plus rice and seaweed. Check, check, and check. The wasabi and ginger that come alongside sushi are low-FODMAP ingredients; if you're gluten-free you'll also want to bring packets of gluten-free tamari or soy sauce. You can also mix things up and order sashimi (just the fish) or sushi pieces (those are the slabs of fish on top of mounds of rice). Just beware of fancy rolls like "crunchy" or "spicy" ones, or those with lots of avocado or sauces (like eel often does), because it's harder to tell what you're getting. Sushi appetizers, sadly, are no-nos—gyoza dumplings are wrapped in wheat-flour-based covers; edamame soybeans are high in galacto-oligosaccharides and fructans; miso soup itself hasn't been tested but is usually made with scallions, which (unless they only use the green parts) are also off-limits.

Chinese: The sauces often used in Chinese stir-fries and other dishes can be hard to decipher in terms of what's in them; wheat-containing soy sauce is a central ingredient to many recipes and may put you over your limit if used in excess. Many Chinese restaurants, however, offer "diet" menus that feature vegetables, meat, seafood, and tofu that's been steamed, usually served with the sauce on the side. You can easily order off this menu as long as you make sure the veggies are ones you can have—any kind of meat or seafood with green beans, carrots, bean sprouts, bok choy, zucchini, or broccoli, for instance (you may be OK if you pick any onions out of a stir-fry, but you're better off being up front about your needs and avoiding them altogether). Flavor it

with up to 2 tablespoons soy sauce and a side of brown or white rice—just skip those little packets of duck sauce, which are often made with off-limits high-fructose corn syrup and apricots.

Thai: Because Thai food is similar to Chinese, you'll find some of the same pros and cons. But with even more dishes revolving around rice and rice-based ingredients like noodles and spring roll wrappers, you'll likely be able to find something at a Thai restaurant that works for you—with a little tweaking. Pad Thai, the staple Thai noodle dish, can be fine if it's prepared with no garlic, onion, or mystery sauce (it's wise to ask the chef to leave out any premade sauces or curries as well, because it's tough to know exactly what's in them). Fresh vegetable spring rolls usually contain just small amounts of low-FODMAP vegetables, herbs, rice noodle wrappers, and tofu or shrimp; just ask what's in the peanut sauce (which is less likely to work) before you dip. And your server can likely help you tweak any stir-fry dish to make sure the ingredients are safe. My local Thai place can do a simple-but-safe stir-fry with zucchini, carrots, bell peppers, and chicken; you can also ask for a fried rice

# Low-FODMAP Fast Food

Because orders are standardized at most casual chain restaurants, it can be hard to eliminate offending ingredients. However, with some careful consideration, there are some options using low-FODMAP ingredients that will work for phase one of the Go Low plan. Here are some you can try:

**CHIPOTLE:** Soft or crunchy tacos with brown or white rice, carnitas, cheese, and romaine lettuce (sadly, the barbacoa, chicken, and tofu sofritas options are all made with garlic, as is—sniffle, sniffle—the guacamole); burrito bowl with rice, carnitas, cheese, and romaine lettuce; cheese quesadilla on corn tortilla with carnitas (kids' menu). You can also have any of these options with no meat at all.

**JIMMY JOHN'S:** JJ Unwiches (sandwiches wrapped in lettuce leaves) including the Turkey Tom, Big John (roast beef), and Club Lulu (turkey and bacon)

**PANERA BREAD:** Caesar Salad (no croutons, no dressing), Seasonal Greens Salad (no onions, no dressing), Greek Salad (no onions, no dressing)

**WENDY'S:** Plain baked potato, Garden Salad (no dressing or croutons)

**WAFFLE HOUSE:** 2 eggs with a side of bacon

**IN-N-OUT BURGER:** Hamburger Protein Style, no sauce or onions + french fries

**STARBUCKS:** Protein Bistro Box (eat just the hard-boiled egg, cheddar cheese, and grapes); fruit cup (leave out any high-FODMAP fruits like apples, but grapes, most melon, and most berries are all OK to eat); oatmeal cup with fresh blueberries and/or brown sugar; Chewy Chocolate Cookie. Note: Starbucks stocks lactose-free milk, but using it won't make all drinks low FODMAP or even lactose-free, for that matter, because the mixes for fancy drinks like caramel lattes and light Frappuccinos contain dairy. Be sure to ask the ingredients before you order, and stick with something without added flavoring, like a latte with lactose-free milk.

dish to be customized to your needs (for instance, no onions/garlic—just rice, carrots, bell peppers, water chestnuts, chicken, beef, shrimp, tofu, Thai basil, peanuts, soy sauce, and/or lime).

**Mexican:** Featuring loads of beans, cheese, and avocado, not to mention the strong flavors of onion and garlic, Mexican food can be tough to navigate. Depending on how the meats are seasoned, you might be able to put together a meal with one of those meats at the center. Shrimp or fish might be a good option, because if it's prepared to order, you can ask for it to be cooked without seasonings. Because you can likely eat a handful of items on the salads and side dishes section of the menu, it may make sense to order from there and piece together your own meal. Try ordering a salad with grilled (plain) chicken or shrimp along with a side of two corn tortillas and some unseasoned rice, to make your own little chicken wraps.

**Indian:** Another challenging cuisine, Indian food often contains beans like lentils and chickpeas in large amounts, sauces that contain onion and cream, and puffy wheat-laden breads. Rice, as long as it's prepared with no onions,

garlic, or peas (as is sometimes the case at Indian restaurants), is one safe food. If the restaurant you're at has a Jain menu, that's a good place for you to start— people who follow the dietary customs of this religion don't eat anything it considers living, including plants that grow underground, like onions and garlic. Honey is also forbidden. So an okra or eggplant dish on a Jain menu with a side of rice, for instance, might be suitable for you. Indian restaurants may be best saved for later in your Go Low journey, when you've reintroduced the various FODMAP varieties and can ease up on some of the restrictions of Go Low phase one; however, if you find yourself at an Indian restaurant during this early phase, be sure to ask lots of questions and don't be afraid to ask that the chef prepare something plain for you.

**Greek:** Mediterranean cuisines like Greek, Lebanese, Israeli, and more can be a challenge because beans like chickpeas are central to many meals. The light and simple nature of Mediterranean food, however, means you have a good base of ingredients to work with—and using them, you can likely build a meal that will be suitable for you. A Greek salad, for instance—hold the onions, use oil and lemon juice as dressing—can fit in beautifully. Grilled chicken, lamb, fish, or shrimp can be wonderful entrées with a side dish of roasted lemon potatoes or rice—as long as it's all prepared without onions or garlic.

Diner: The food at diners is typically fast, simple, and made to order, making this sort of restaurant perfect if you have to eat out when you Go Low. Tell the server up front that you need your food prepared with no seasonings—onions and garlic included. Then go ahead and order some steak with a baked potato and green beans, or grilled chicken with fries and a salad. A Greek salad (hold the onions), Caesar salad with grilled chicken or shrimp (hold the croutons), or Cobb salad (just watch to make sure you're eating no more than an eighth of an avocado) are all great choices if you use oil and lemon juice or a bit of vinegar for your dressing. Burgers are often made with chopped onions, so be wary of ordering them. But the biggest reason diners are the best: all-day breakfast. Sunny-side-up eggs; a spinach, tomato, and feta omelet; or a cheddar omelet with home fries (provided the home fries are not made with onions—if so, get the regular fries instead) are perfect options at any hour. Yay for diners!

Steak house: These restaurants are great options for low-FODMAP diners, whether they like steak or not. The reason? Simplicity. You can't go wrong with a piece of broiled or grilled meat or fish, a medium baked potato with a teaspoon of butter, and a side of sautéed spinach or a garden salad with oil and vinegar. (OK, OK, it's possible to mess up here, too—as always, talk to your server to make sure your order is prepared without garlic and onion or any other surprise seasonings.)

## Dining Hall Lowdown

Going Low in either high school or college can be tough—the lack of acceptable food choices combined with a crazy schedule and friends who live on pizza make things difficult enough that I've dedicated an entire section (on page 101) to how to figure out what your cafeteria or dining hall serves and what to do about it. But despite the real challenges, Going Low in a college cafeteria—or being on any restrictive diet, for that matter—is easier now than ever. That's because of the level of transparency that currently exists in university food service. In years past, it was hard for a student to find out what ingredients were used in preparing the foods they picked up at the

# Dorm Room Delicacies

You can get creative in the dining hall, and undoubtedly you will. But supplementing clever cafeteria hacks with foods you can pick up at the school convenience store or local grocery will help you make doing the Go Low plan on campus a reality. You may have only a mini fridge and a microwave down the hall, but you can accomplish a lot more than you think. Here are a few foods to keep on hand that work especially well for teensy fridges and tight quarters with little cooking capability:

- Go Low–approved nuts (walnuts, peanuts, pecans)
- Lactose-free yogurt
- Go Low–approved cereal (including EnviroKidz Gorilla Munch and Peanut Butter Panda Puffs, Erewhon Corn Flakes and Crispy Brown Rice)
- Go Low–approved milk or milk alternative (lactose-free milk, unsweetened almond milk)
- Individual packets of Go Low–approved oatmeal or oatmeal cups (like Nature's Path or Quaker plain)

- Go Low–approved cheese
- Go Low–approved on-the-go meal/snack drink like ProNourish Low FODMAP Nutritional Drink
- Go Low–approved microwave popcorn (like Quinn)
- Go Low–approved snack bars (try Nature Valley crunchy peanut butter/cinnamon granola bars and Be Nice low-FODMAP bars, available online)

cafeteria. Nowadays, many university food-service operations have websites dedicated to providing students with this very information. With increases in the incidence of food allergies and sensitivities, dietary preferences like vegetarianism and veganism, and heightened general awareness about health and sustainability, students are demanding to know what is in their food, and sometimes even where it comes from—and food-service companies and schools are obliging. In the next chapter, I'll give you some strategies for finding out what, exactly, your college dining hall puts in their food—and how you might be able to change it. Then, once you've done your homework, it's time to eat!

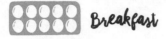 **Breakfast**

- Cheerios with lactose-free milk or unsweetened almond milk and blueberries
- Eggs prepared at the grill any style (make sure scrambled eggs don't have milk added) + a small banana

- 2 hard-boiled eggs + ½ grapefruit sprinkled with ½ teaspoon sugar
- ½ cup (115 g) oatmeal topped with 5 medium (70 g) strawberries, chopped; 1 tablespoon walnut pieces; and 1 teaspoon maple syrup

**Lunch**

- Baked potato sprinkled with ¼ cup (25 g) cheddar and ½ cup (20 g) spinach or other Go Low veggies (from the salad bar if necessary)
- Salad with 1 cup (35 g) romaine, 3 ounces (85 g) grilled chicken, ¼ cup (30 g) cucumber, ½ cup (75 g) quinoa, 2 tablespoons sliced olives, topped with 1 tablespoon olive oil and 1 teaspoon lemon juice

- Breadless turkey breast sandwich made with 2 slices of turkey, 1 slice of tomato, and up to 2 tablespoons mayo between 2 leaves of romaine lettuce + a side of potato chips

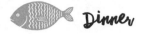

# Dinner

- DIY rice bowl (cobble together the hot meal options and the salad bar): 1 cup (40 g) baby spinach topped with 1 cup (180 g) hot brown or white rice, ¼ cup (35 g) raw zucchini, ¼ cup (30 g) raw carrots, ⅓ cup (80 g) cubed firm tofu, 2 teaspoons peanuts, a sprinkle of cilantro, olive oil, and rice wine vinegar

- DIY quinoa bowl (this one can be done strictly at the salad bar): 1 cup (155 g) quinoa, ¼ cup (25 g) red bell peppers, 1 hard-boiled egg, ¼ cup (55 g) tuna, 1 teaspoon sunflower seeds, 1 tablespoon oil, 1 teaspoon apple cider vinegar

- Angelic deviled eggs: Liberate 2 hard-boiled eggs from the salad bar. Cut in half, remove the yolks, and mix with a little bit of mayonnaise and mustard. Season with salt and pepper, then stuff the filling back into the egg halves. Voilà! Serve with a side salad and some rice or quinoa.

- Chicken with satay sauce: Bring your own gluten-free tamari packets. Put 2 tablespoons of peanut butter in a microwave-safe bowl and heat gently until the peanut butter softens. Add tamari and crushed red pepper (usually available at the pizza station). Microwave again for a few seconds to meld flavors, and mix again. Thin with water as needed. Serve alongside plain grilled chicken, spinach, and rice.

# Sneaky Sources of FODMAPs

If only FODMAPs wore a big sign on them that said "Don't eat me (for now)." All too often, they're camouflaged in dishes and easy to miss. Here are some places where they're likely to be lurking:

**SALAD DRESSINGS:** Store-bought salad dressings are often made with high-fructose corn syrup; fresh may have buttermilk or sour cream—and all are likely to contain some minced onion or garlic. Opt for olive oil mixed with lemon juice, red wine vinegar, or rice wine vinegar instead (balsamic vinegar can have excess fructose).

**SOUPS:** Mirepoix—sautéed carrots, onion, and celery—is routinely used as a base for soup broth. What's more, many recipes add cream or milk—bottom line, most restaurant-prepared soups are a no-go for you (see Chapter 9 for recipes for easy soups you can make at home, though).

**BURGERS (HAMBURGERS, TURKEY BURGERS, SALMON BURGERS, VEGGIE BURGERS, ETC.):** Many chefs and home cooks mix in finely chopped onions and seasonings like garlic powder. Some, however, are safe—it's smart to ask before you eat. Also specify that you don't want your burger seasoned, as many chefs add garlic or onion powder before the patty goes on the grill.

**SAUCES:** You probably know that finding an Italian restaurant that doesn't use garlic and onions in its tomato sauce is about as easy as finding a gossip site without pictures of some celeb's sideboob. But did you know that plenty of other standard sauces, like Thai green curry or Indian masala, use them as well? Like soups, many sauces also use thickeners that aren't low-FODMAP friendly. It's best, for now, to avoid sauces—unless you're 100 percent sure that they're made with low-FODMAP ingredients.

## THE SALAD BAR

One option in most college cafeterias that can be your best friend is the salad bar. It's easy to build a salad that works on the Go Low plan. Here's a six-step plan to help you build a low-FODMAP salad:

**1.** *Go green:* Start with any leaf of your choice, for example, romaine lettuce, iceberg lettuce, spinach, arugula, mesclun, or kale.

**2.** *Combine some colors:* Add up to 1¼ cups (roughly 100 g) total of two to four low-FODMAP vegetables, such as cucumbers, carrots, red cabbage, tomatoes, bell peppers, zucchini, fennel, or yellow squash.

**3.** *Add carbs or crunch:* Add texture and keep it interesting by sprinkling on ½ cup (75 g) of a fiber-rich grain like quinoa, brown rice, or wild rice or 1 tablespoon of a crunchy nut like walnuts, pine nuts, pecans, or peanuts.

**4.** *Pick your protein:* Protein is crucial to creating a salad that feels like a meal (and keeps you energized until dinner). Salad bars often have plain cooked proteins; just make sure they're cooked using only low-FODMAP

ingredients (no onion or garlic!) and choose your Go Low–approved favorite, such as grilled chicken, hard-boiled egg, cubed tofu, feta, cheddar, or (nonbreaded) shrimp.

**5.** *Dress it:* Some store-bought salad dressings are fine for a low-FODMAP plan, but you often can't tell what's in the dressing at a salad bar. Instead, play it safe and dress your salad with 1 tablespoon olive oil and 1 teaspoon lemon juice, apple cider vinegar, or rice wine vinegar. (Or, if you can, make the yummy dressing for my Rainbow Mason Jar Salad on page 163 and bring from home.)

**6.** *Make it extra special:* A sprinkle of a low-FODMAP ingredient like bacon (make sure it's really bacon and not fake bacon bits), grated Parmesan, olives, sliced grapes, orange segments, or a fresh herb like cilantro or basil can take your salad to the next level. Add as needed for flavor and fun.

And don't forget, the salad bar is good for more than just salads. Think of the items on the salad bar as ingredients that the cafeteria staff have kindly cleaned, washed, cut, and in some cases even cooked for you (thank you, weird cafeteria dude who always wants to talk about the football team!) so you can hack any cafeteria offering into a meal. For example: If the hot meal offered is rotisserie chicken made with onion powder and garlic powder, you know that you can't get the chicken (boo). But you can ask for the steamed zucchini and rice that come on the side and bring them over to the salad bar for a makeover. Drizzle on 1 tablespoon olive oil and 1 teaspoon lemon juice, add a little plain grilled chicken and sliced olives, and suddenly you've got a meal.

Warning: If your cafeteria is the type where a cashier rings up your food after you've gathered it, this "hack the caf" method might drive the poor cafeteria worker crazy. But she'll figure out a way to charge your card—and it's a small price to pay for finding a way to make the dining hall work for you.

I've scoured a sampling of college cafeteria menus from around the country to create a list of possible go-to dining hall meals for you on pages 78 and 79.

# CHAPTER 5

## The Plan:

## ELIMINATION AND REINTRODUCTION

In Chapter 4, I made it clear that low-FODMAP eating is not meant to be forever. This chapter will walk you through the two phases of the program: phase one, the two- to six-week elimination round, and phase two, when you will begin to reintroduce some of the foods you've removed to find out what you can tolerate.

### GO LOW PHASE ONE: THE ELIMINATION ROUND

Commit to the plan by eating nothing but Go foods for two to six weeks. Lists of the foods you can eat and the amounts that are OK during this phase begin on page 55. You can also include Slow foods, as long as you proceed with extreme caution and take extra care to keep the portion sizes small. Sound hard? Well, there's no doubt that it's a challenge. But you can also consider it an adventure. It's kind of like going away to summer camp. So you have to take a break from Snapchat for a few weeks. But, you know it will be there waiting for you when you get back—and in its absence, you may discover some cool things along the way (like real live friends! Or, in the case of the Go Low plan, lactose-free yogurt!).

Your favorite foods, too, will still be there when you finish up phase one of the Go Low plan—but I'll give you so many delicious ideas that, guaranteed, you'll want to continue eating them after you're long done with this stage. Not to mention, eating these low-FODMAP foods just may get you feeling better, which will motivate and inspire you to stick with it.

Easy peasy, right? You probably read through the delicious-sounding meal and snack options in Chapter 4 and didn't even notice that garlic, hummus, ice cream, and bagels are off-limits. Er, you did? OK, well, here's my advice: Focus on what you *can* eat, and the foods you can't have will fade into the distance. And for those moments when you can't

simply forget what you're missing out on, remind yourself that this is temporary and that the goal is not for you to be miserable but for you to feel great.

If it feels like a lot, fear not—as soon as this initial phase is over, we won't waste any time getting you to experiment with No foods to see what you can tolerate. In the meantime, try something different, like my Chocolate-Covered Strawberry Shake (page 183) or Happy Belly Breakfast Tacos (page 149), or ask your parent to pick up a new-to-you low-FODMAP food like star fruit at the exotic fruit market. Making it fun helps you stick with it so you can finally get the relief you deserve.

---

TRY THIS

## Dear Diary

When you begin the Go Low FODMAP challenge, it's super important that you keep a detailed journal of what you're eating and how you feel—just as it was important to keep a journal of your symptoms when you were preparing to see your doctor (see page 13). The reason: Taking notes not only will help you stay honest about what you're eating but will also help you pinpoint what's affecting you and how. On the next page is an example of what you should track; I recommend buying a small notebook dedicated just for this purpose so all of your records are in one place (also, it's a great excuse to buy a cool notebook like the ones at poppin.com). You can also download a food journal app like MyFitnessPal.

# GO LOW PHASE TWO: THE NO CHALLENGE

Once you've lived Go Low phase one, the elimination for two to six weeks, and have found relief from your symptoms (I hope!), it's time to test the higher-FODMAP foods so you can expand your eating options. Remember, it's not that you can never eat FODMAP-containing foods again—you just need to make sure you're not eating too much of the ones that put you over the edge. All it takes is a little experimentation and patience to figure out how to enjoy some of the foods you're missing without retriggering those nasty symptoms.

Take phase two, the No Challenge, one step at a time. Once you've found relief from your symptoms during phase one of Going Low, you can rest there for a few weeks and enjoy feeling good. But by week six, it's time to begin experimenting. As soon as you feel you're ready, here's how it works.

## Step One: Pick a FODMAP, Any FODMAP

Choose one class of FODMAPs to experiment with (this isn't a pop quiz—you can refresh your memory by taking a look at page 43). Try one typical serving of a food that's high in that class

of FODMAP and that class of FODMAP only—your best bet is to stick with the challenge foods that I've suggested on page 88.

## Step Two: Test It Out

Step two is a three-day test. Here's what you'll do:

Day 1: Add a food containing the FODMAP you've decided to experiment with to only one meal, in the amount recommended. Feeling good? Great. Now, sleep on it and see how you feel the next morning. Still good? Great.

Day 2: Have the same food again—this time, double the amount you ate yesterday. Still feeling good? Awesome!

Day 3: If you're still in good shape, eat the food once again in the same amount you had on day 2. Doesn't seem to bother you? Then you're in the clear with this food and can include it in your diet in moderate amounts.

If at any point during this trial period you begin to experience symptoms again, simply drop the new food and skip immediately to step three, eating just a baseline Go Low diet for three or more days, until you feel better.

## Step Three: **Back to Basics**

For step three, go back to your baseline diet—in other words, eat only what's OK during Go Low phase one and don't eat any of the newly introduced foods—for three days. Even though you ruled out the food that you just tried as something that's giving you major problems, there's still some fine-tuning to do here—for instance, you may tolerate small amounts of dairy and beans on their own, but not at the same meal. So to get the best picture of how your body handles each FODMAP individually, you'll want to go back to your basic diet before you test a new food.

## Step Four: **Replay**

Now, pick a new food to try, and start with step one all over again!

Remember: During the No Challenge, you want to introduce as many foods as possible to give your diet the most variety and stick-with-it-ability (that's a technical term). However, the object is getting you well. If you start to experience symptoms after introducing any new food, don't push it. Put it on the

| TIME | FOOD | SYMPTOMS | NOTES |
|------|------|----------|-------|
| 2:00 p.m. | Lactose-free cheese stick; 3 strawberries | Stomach felt a little queasy | Was feeling stressed out before SAT prep class |
| 6:00 p.m. | Omelet with spinach and tomato and gluten-free toast | None | Eating with family, having a nice time |
| | | | |
| | | | |

| TIME | FOOD | SYMPTOMS | NOTES |
|------|------|----------|-------|
|      |      |          |       |
|      |      |          |       |
|      |      |          |       |
|      |      |          |       |
|      |      |          |       |
|      |      |          |       |
|      |      |          |       |
|      |      |          |       |

## GETTING STARTED ON A RESTRICTED DIET

"It's really hard at first, and you may be tempted to eat something that isn't necessarily good for you. But just know that it won't do you any good."

"Remember that sometimes food is just fuel."

"Once you get used to the diet, it isn't as difficult as it seems."

"Eating something that you know will upset your stomach is not worth it!"

"Stay strong. Read all labels."

back burner—you can always revisit it in different amounts later on in the process.

So let's say you want to start with fructose. A good food to challenge with would be honey. Add a serving of honey—1 teaspoon—to a cup of approved herbal tea or plain lactose-free yogurt on day one. No symptoms? Great. On day two, do the same thing, but this time with 2 teaspoons. If all is well, on day three have the same, 2 teaspoons. If you continue to feel good, you now know that fructose (in moderation) is not your problem. Unpleasant symptoms? We have a culprit. You can stop here and go back to your baseline diet. Three or more days later, when you're feeling well again, test out a different FODMAP.

## THE BEST CHALLENGE FOODS

Because many high-FODMAP foods contain a combination of FODMAPs, use the foods in the table on page 90 as your challenge foods—this way you'll more easily pinpoint which FODMAP is giving you the trouble.

## FAQS ABOUT REINTRODUCTION

### What Food Should I Start With?

The one you miss the most—although don't get too excited; you're going to have to wait until you've completed testing each class of foods before you can begin eating it regularly again (if all goes well).

## Does It Matter When I Eat the Food?

Yes. There's no right time of day to reintroduce a food, but do try to do it earlier rather than later—with breakfast or lunch, or at latest an afternoon snack—so that you won't snooze through any symptoms.

If you eat a late dinner with your first clove of garlic in six weeks and then head straight to bed, you might be deep in slumber when gas and bloating hit. And granted, if you're sleeping through symptoms, they may not be

that bad; however, for the purpose of exploration, it probably makes sense to be conscious when you're most likely to feel something, right?

## Do I Need to Eat the Challenge Food in the Same Form Each Time?

Yes—it won't hurt your experiment to do so, and it just might help you get to the bottom of things. If you have a cup of tea with honey in it on day one, a smoothie on day two, and a bowl of oatmeal on day three, it will be harder to tell what's causing your symptoms in the event that you start feeling unwell. Try to have the same food three days in a row in the same way, preferably along with a food you've

| FODMAP | DAY ONE | DAY TWO + DAY THREE |
| --- | --- | --- |
| Fructo-oligosaccharides (FOS), vegetables | ½ clove garlic | 1 clove garlic |
| Fructo-oligosaccharides (FOS), grains | 1 slice of wheat bread | 2 slices of wheat bread |
| Galacto-oligosaccharides (GOS) | ¼ cup (50 g) canned kidney beans | ½ cup (100 g) canned kidney beans |
| Polyols (mannitol) | ¼ cup (18 g) button mushrooms | ½ cup (35 g) button mushrooms |
| Polyols (sorbitol) | 1 medium apricot or 3 blackberries | 2 medium apricots or 6 blackberries |
| Lactose | ½ cup (120 ml) milk | 1 cup (240 ml) milk |
| Fructose | 1 teaspoon honey | 2 teaspoons honey |

eaten regularly with no problem while on the Go Low plan—honey in a 3-ounce (85 g) serving of lactose-free yogurt, for instance. Minimizing the number of variables will help you easily identify the causes of your tummy troubles.

## I'm Excited to Try the Foods I've Been Missing. Is It OK If I Go Out to Eat and Celebrate with a Big Bowl of Real-Deal Wheat Pasta (Pasta!!) or a Plate of Onion Rings (Onions!!)?

Sad to say, but, no. Because portion size matters, it's crucial that you test out foods in moderate amounts to see what you can tolerate. To do that, you need full control in the kitchen. A bowl of pasta at a restaurant is way too big and too likely to cause symptoms to get a handle on what you might be able to eat. Onion rings, delicious though they are, are also battered with flour and drenched in oil—adding several new variables that you might react to. Stay home (for now), and keep it simple.

## How Do I Retest a FODMAP That Didn't Go Well the First Time I Tried?

Try the same food; however, this time you'll want to start with half the amount you started with last time. Experienced gas and bloating from that 1 teaspoon honey? Try ½ teaspoon next time.

Remember, much of your tolerance for FODMAPs depends on portion size—so there's a decent chance you'll find that you're OK with a super small amount. It doesn't sound like much, but it's helpful for you to get a handle on what you can get away with before your gut begins to revolt. FODMAP researchers say it's unlikely that you'll have to completely eliminate a food.

### I'm Feeling Good on the Go Low Plan. Why Risk Messing It Up? Can't I Just Keep Eating This Way Forever?

You really shouldn't. First of all, eating according to the Go Low elimination plan can get boring—sure, I've done everything I can to make it as interesting as possible, but there's no doubt that it's a limited way of eating that can be a burden on your social life and family relationships. But more important, while going on a low-FODMAP diet may diminish your gut symptoms, it may also have a negative impact on your gut microbiome, which isn't good for your overall health, according to research from Australia. FODMAP scientists have said that their results have shown how important it is to ease up on restrictions and vary the diet as much as possible, as soon as possible.

## YOUR LIFE, YOUR PLAN

If you're like most teenagers, the responsibility of shopping for groceries and cooking probably falls on one or both of your parents. Sound familiar? Well, the two to six weeks that you're in phase one of the Go Low plan is a great time to get familiar with how your meal gets from wherever the food came from to landing on your plate. The reason: Just by reading this book, you're becoming your family's resident expert on the low-FODMAP diet. Of course you are! You're the one on the plan, and you need to know the ins and outs of it, wherever you are—no matter how much your parents like to "helicopter" you. Even if they tend to take over when it comes to food, you are the one who will feel better after successfully staying on this plan. Taking ownership over some of the food shopping and prep can ensure that you actually stay on your Go Low plan long enough to reap the benefits.

### Learn to Shop

The simple act of getting food from the farm, warehouse, or store to you is the first crucial step to eating according to the Go Low plan. If your kitchen pantry and refrigerator are packed with products you can eat and ingredients you can easily make, sticking with the plan will be that much easier. Even if you don't typically buy groceries in your house, it's a great idea for you to begin playing a bigger role in acquiring food for yourself and your family as you start phase one of the Go Low plan. Here are a few tips:

Get the app: Going low? Well, there's an app for that, of course. As I mentioned earlier, the team at Monash University offers a smartphone app (iPhone and Android) that features a frequently updated database of the FODMAP content in foods, straight from their laboratory in Melbourne, Australia. A red-, yellow-, or green-light system makes it easy to decipher which foods you can eat. Almonds? Stop right there—that's a red-light food; swap them for pecans and you'll be just fine, however. Zucchini? Green light, go! The app is a

## NOTES

Use this space to keep track of how you feel as you reintroduce No foods and any other relevant information you may uncover. (There are additional notes pages at the back of this book.)

# NOTES

bit pricier than most but is well worth the money.

**Brush up on your (label) reading:** The most important—really the only important—thing you can look at to determine if a food is OK for you to eat is its ingredients label. While most packaged foods in the United States haven't been analyzed for FODMAP content, you can still determine whether a food is likely to be safe by scouring the ingredients list. Not sure about something? Look it up on the Monash University app. To save you some trouble, take a look at the packaged-food ingredients list on page 61 for some red flags.

**Select a nutrition-minded store:** Low-FODMAP ingredients and products are everywhere. But stores that have a good selection of gluten-free, Paleo, and other health-focused foods may give you a wider array of options. You still have to read labels (see "Gluten-Free Does Not Equal Low FODMAP" on page 60), but a store that makes an effort to stock items that fit into specialized diets can be a good place to start. You can also seek out conventional grocery chains that have an RDN on staff, like H-E-B, Safeway, ShopRite, Kroger, Giant

Eagle, Bashas', and Hy-Vee. The reason? These health-and-nutrition-focused professionals are trained in special diets; RDNs who work in grocery stores are pros at helping people track down the right foods for them. You can knock on their window and ask for some help— think of them like your own in-store personal shoppers!

**Go Low online:** I love online grocery shopping for two reasons: One, timing becomes a nonissue. In other words, if your dad does the weekly grocery run while you're at volleyball practice, you can still participate. Two, you can take your time looking at ingredients lists and figuring out the foods that will work best for you. And three, you can do it all from the same device you just binge watched *Empire* on—all while sending your BFF snaps of you as a dog. Online grocery options vary by region; however, services like Thrive Market (thrivemarket.com) and AmazonFresh (fresh.amazon.com) are available around the country and give you access to a lot of great foods.

## Conquer the Kitchen

Maybe you're not much of a chef—yet. But now is as good a time as any to acquire some culinary skills or at least help your parents out enough to start getting a feel for things. Bonus: Being confident and skilled in the kitchen will enable you to be healthier for life (also it's a great way to save money and make friends—who doesn't love a delicious home-cooked meal?!).

**Whet your appetite:** Being a cooking enthusiast is a great first step to getting comfortable in the kitchen. Watch the Food Network, *Top Chef*, or YouTube channels like Tasty. Read food magazines and blogs. You'll be surprised by how much you learn and inspired by just watching.

**Sign up for a cooking class:** If your school offers classes that take place in a kitchen, take one. If not—or your schedule is already too packed—look into taking a class or two in your free time. Local schools in your area may offer cooking classes just for teens; culinary-supply chain stores like Sur La Table and Williams-Sonoma also offer specialized courses in some locations. You may also want to Google "low-FODMAP cooking class" and your hometown or closest city—more and more RDNs and chefs are offering low-FODMAP cooking classes; if you're lucky enough to find one, I recommend

participating with a parent so you can both learn and explore low-FODMAP foods at the same time and make it a fun expedition to go on together.

**Make a meal plan:** If you're not quite ready to whip up dinner for your whole family, that's OK. Start by scribbling down some notes. What Go Low–approved breakfasts do you think you might want each day? And which Go Low dinners would your whole family eat? Put together a list and share it with the person in your family who does the cooking; helping make decisions about what the people in your house will eat is a great first step to owning the kitchen.

**Play the role of sous chef:** In a professional kitchen, the sous chef is the second-in-command. Ask the head chef in your home, whether it's Mom, Dad, or someone else, if you can play the role of assistant for the day; this will help you get your feet wet and gain proficiency in the kitchen before taking the reins yourself.

**Do it yourself:** Cooking is kind of like learning a foreign language. You can learn a lot from studying and watching other people hone their skills. But you won't master it until you start putting the knowledge you've gained into practice. Ask the person in charge of your family's kitchen if you can plan and prepare one meal. Choose something simple so your first effort goes as smoothly as possible. If that goes well, see if you can make it a regular occurrence. You're not a kid, of course, but you might be down with a campaign called Kids Cook Monday, which inspires families to get young people in the kitchen one day a week. Check out thekidscookmonday.org for ideas on easy ways to get started.

## Think Ahead

Thinking ahead is also crucial to your Go Low success. If you're always scrambling at the last minute to figure out what to eat, you're more likely to grab the wrong thing in a hurry. Instead, make like a Boy Scout and "be prepared." Here are a few ways you can do just that, supported by the great groceries you picked up.

**Set yourself up with grab-and-go breakfasts:** Ah, breakfast. It's the most important meal of the day (so says your mom—and loads of nutrition experts, it turns out) and, somehow, the hardest to make time for. Think ahead about what you might eat for your morning meal— Go Low–approved smoothies, cereals,

yogurts, and egg-based dishes can all be great choices (see page 146 for breakfast recipes). However, they're not always conducive to those mornings when you just need to get going. So be prepared (and practical) with foods you can eat on the run. See "Breakfasts on the Run" on page 97 for some ideas.

**Stock up on snacks:** How many times a day do you eat a snack? If you grab a nosh more times a day than you pause for a meal, you're not alone—American teenagers now eat an average of almost four snacks per day, according to research firm NPD Group. And because many of the foods we may reach for when it's snack time, such as pretzels, energy bars, apples, and cookies, are not typically Go Low approved, snack time can be an extra challenge. Make sure to keep Go Low snacks like gluten-free pretzels or popcorn on hand. (For more ideas see "Go Low Snacks" on page 64.)

**Have backup meals ready to go:** It's great if you can cook for your family. And it's equally wonderful if your parents are on board and willing to make the Go Low–approved meals for everyone. But being prepared means that you have to be ready for whatever comes your way. And that includes

# Breakfasts on the Run

- Make-it-yourself power packs. Get a bunch of ziplock bags, a box of your favorite Go Low–approved cold cereal, and a bag of your favorite Go Low–approved nuts or seeds. Scoop one serving of cereal and one serving of nuts or seeds into each bag. And there you have it—ready-to-go power packs.

- Single-serving breakfast recipes. Mix up a few days' worth of Easy Peasy Chia Pudding (page 182) or Belly Balancing Overnight Oats (page 153) in small mason jars or glass bowls with lids (like the ones made by Pyrex). It will take a little time, but you'll be glad to have a homemade meal.

- Peanut butter squeeze packs (like Justin's Classic Peanut Butter)

- Bananas

- Single-serving lactose-free yogurts (like the ones by Green Valley Organics)

- Single-serving lactose-free cheese (like Cabot Seriously Sharp Cheddar)

- Hard-boiled eggs

those nights when everyone's running late and Mom wants to order a pizza, or it's your sister's birthday and all she wants is her most favorite meal of honey-cashew chicken with cauliflower in garlic sauce (in other words, no, no, no, and no—sigh).

## GOING LOW IN HIGH SCHOOL

Cafeteria food can be underwhelming enough to begin with. Throw in some dietary restrictions, and it's not surprising if you'd rather swap in advanced calculus for your lunch period. But it doesn't have to be this way! And it won't, once we're finished here.

I need you to promise you will remember these three words: *You require fuel.* With the average start time for public high schools in the United States clocking in at roughly 8:00 AM (meaning many are even earlier), by the time lunchtime rolls around it's likely been a good four, five, maybe even six hours since you last put food in your body. As you'll read in the next chapter, you never want to go more than four or five hours without eating, because doing so can lead to an energy slump that you don't need when you're trying to memorize the quadratic formula. Food = fuel. And by lunch period, you'll need some.

## USING THE BATHROOM AT SCHOOL

"I have a free bathroom pass that my head of year gave me."

"At the beginning of the school year, most classes gave out—at the most—ten bathroom passes that were for the whole year. I knew that wouldn't work out for me at all, so I told my mom and she emailed all of my teachers, telling them that I have GI issues. So I have a free pass in almost every class."

"I have had teachers say I can't go during class."

"[Having enough bathroom passes] was part of my accommodation that was set up in a meeting with Disabilities Services."

"Using the bathroom is always stressful because I have to wait until no one's in there so I can go without anyone hearing."

The second reason lunch is so important is that your brain needs a break. We live in a fast-paced world where many of us have fallen out of the habit of stopping during the day to relax for a few minutes (I'll take the blame for this on behalf of adults, because we were the ones who started this ridiculous trend). If you've ever spent your lunch period shoving a sandwich in your mouth while you finish some homework, you know that failing to take a break can make your day feel long and tiresome—and while it might prevent you from getting a zero for not turning your homework in, it can make the rest of the day kind of a bust. And as we discussed earlier, being stressed can worsen digestive symptoms. It's true: Having a little time to hang out with friends to laugh and relax may actually be therapy for your stomach. So shying away from lunch period—for nutritional and scheduling reasons—is a big no-no.

## IN THE MOOD FOR CAFETERIA FOOD?

Sadly, it can be hard to know what you're getting when you buy food at the caf. Prepared foods can have ingredients that you wouldn't expect. Plain-seeming rice, for instance, might be cooked in chicken broth that contains

# Lunch or Dinner in a Hurry

Here are a few extra-simple go-to meals you can whip up in a hurry (yes, pouring food in a bowl counts as "whipping up." This isn't *MasterChef Junior*—it's survival!).

- A tuna sandwich made with toasted Go Low–approved gluten-free bread, 1 small can of water-packed chunk light tuna mixed with up to 2 tablespoons mayonnaise, lettuce, and sliced cucumber

- A yogurt parfait: 1 container (6 ounces/ 170 g) lactose-free yogurt topped with 20 (30 g) blueberries and ¾ cup (30 g) EnviroKidz Gorilla Munch Cereal

- Summer pasta: 1 cup (145 g) Go Low–approved gluten-free pasta with 1 teaspoon olive oil, 1 cup (40 g) baby spinach, 1 small (120 g) chopped tomato, and 2 tablespoons shredded Parmesan

- A quinoa bowl made with 1 cup (155 g) prepared quinoa, 2 tablespoons chopped walnuts, ½ cup (75 g) sliced red grapes, and flaked canned salmon or (if there's some leftover in the fridge) grilled chicken

onions. Sautéed vegetables very well might have garlic in them. What's more, most school cafeterias these days don't make their food from scratch—in other words, food comes to them preprepared from a factory or commissary kitchen (a main facility where all of the cooking is done before it's sent out to your school). The servers at your school might not even know what's in the foods they're plopping onto plates!

So what's the lesson here? Well, simple. If you want to eat in a cafeteria and stick with a low-FODMAP plan, it's crucial that you ask questions and get answers. You might not always get the answers you need—but you won't know until you try. In the end, your ability to Go Low in your school cafeteria will really depend on the cafeteria itself, including how food is prepared and how much information the people who work there can give you.

## How to Be a Lunch-Period Private Eye

To get to the bottom of what's in the foods at your cafeteria, your best bet is to track down the person who holds this crucial information. Here's a simple three-step strategy you can use to get the information you need:

## STAYING ON A RESTRICTED DIET

"I'm able to stick with it because I'm afraid of getting bad stomachaches and having to run to the bathroom, especially when I'm not home."

"If I go off the diet for a few days, my symptoms tend to get a lot worse, so I'd rather avoid that."

"I'm used to it now; it becomes a habit."

"Feeling better encourages me to stick with it."

"Knowing I won't shit my pants has motivated me to stick with it!"

**1.** Arrive in the cafeteria and scope out what you think some good options might be, thinking about what you want to ask about.

**2.** Speak with a friendly server or other caf staffer. Explain to her that you have some food sensitivities and you need to find out what's in some of the foods to know what's safe for you to eat. Chances are, she'll direct you to the chef or the food-service director, who can better address your concerns.

**3.** Say hello to your friendly (I hope!) food-service director, chef, or other knowledgeable person! Not sure what to say? Of course not—it can be tough to speak up for yourself,

especially when it comes to something complicated like going low FODMAP. Here's a sample script of what you can say: "Hi, I'm on a special diet recommended by my registered dietitian and/or doctor called low-FODMAP because I have a sensitivity to certain types of carbohydrates found in different foods. The list of ingredients I can't eat is long, and it's not always easy to tell if prepared foods contain them—so I need your help to figure out what I can eat because you're the one who knows what's in the food here. For example, I can't eat anything with wheat, onions, or garlic in it—even garlic or onion powder. The more simply something is prepared, the better. I noticed chicken,

## Ready-to-Go Go Low

Here are some Go Low–approved foods that are often found in school cafeterias (remember, these foods haven't been tested themselves, but the ingredients and controlled portion sizes should make them a safe bet; remember to always double-check ingredients).

- Nature Valley crunchy granola bars (peanut butter, cinnamon)
- Popcorn Indiana Kettlecorn
- Plain potato chips
- Popchips, sea salt flavor
- Popcorners, Salt of the Earth flavor
- Plain tortilla chips

rice, and sautéed zucchini are being served today. That would be perfect for me, as long as they weren't made with any ingredients on my 'do not eat' list. Can you possibly tell me all of the ingredients that were used?"

## Stay Safe: Brown-Bag It

Your surest bet when eating at the school caf is bringing lunch from home. The main reason, of course, is that you get to control what goes into it and can make it both Go Low–approved and delicious. But there are some other major advantages. High school students who bring lunch from home are more likely to eat nutritious foods over the course of the day, according to a study published in the *American Journal of Health Promotion* (same for eating

breakfast and having dinner as a family, for the record). Depending on what you typically bring from home, you might be able to pack the same lunch with a little tweaking to make it low FODMAP (like swapping your normal bread for a Go Low–approved one). Among the recipes in the back of the book, you will find a number of lunch options that work well on the go; find more toss-in-your-bag school-ready options above.

## GOING LOW IN COLLEGE

If you're in college, the challenges of Going Low are similar to those of someone eating in a high school cafeteria times three, because you might be eating all of your meals in the dining hall—a social experiment designed by adults to turn kids into

# WHAT I WISH MY TEACHERS KNEW

"That you can't just suck it up."

"How my life has changed and how overwhelming it is."

"That it may not be life threatening, but it does affect my ability to concentrate or even stay in class."

"To stop asking kids, 'Is it an emergency?' As a kid I was too embarrassed to answer yes in front of my whole class."

"That it's not just an excuse to get out of class."

people who really, really want to cook for themselves (anything is better than Sunday Surprise!). Plus, you likely don't have a full kitchen in which to make homemade meals to supplement the dining hall food. If this sounds like you, you might want to consider holding off trying Go Low phase one until you're home from school on winter break or for the summer, so you can have slightly more control over what you're eating.

If you're really ready to go and can't wait any longer, it can be done, no doubt—but it will take a little effort and resilience on your part (of course, that's true any time you undertake a low-FODMAP plan). Go you, perseverant person, for accepting the challenge!

Hopping on the Low-FODMAP Express while you're living at school means communication is even more important. Get on a first-name basis with the person who runs the show in your cafeteria—the food-service director, chef, or someone else—to find out what meals are truly safe for you. And don't hesitate to give your input or ask for things you don't see. Maybe they can start to keep some unsweetened almond milk on hand if they don't already—undoubtedly the many lactose-intolerant and vegan students would be thrilled to see it, too.

First, do a little research on what foods your school's dining hall *does* have. Google the name of your school

## FRIENDS, DATING, AND BEING SOCIAL

"I have lost friends. I'm not able to date either."

"It's made me avoid people and become quite antisocial. I get really anxious around people and crowds. I push people away and I tend to be quite awkward."

"People ask me to go out to eat all the time and I would have to say no because of my dietary restrictions and since I did not always feel well."

"Sometimes I can't see my boyfriend because I'm in too much pain or have fear I'm going to fart or poop."

"It can be uncomfortable to tell a friend I can't eat their food."

"Last semester, I was a lot less social because I was sick most of the time."

"My closest friendships have not been affected."

"It's harder to make plans because I don't know how I will be feeling that day."

"My boyfriend is very supportive because he suffers from IBS, too!"

and the phrase "food service" or "dining services." You'll most likely pull up a page that tells you what's on the menu each day at each dining hall and restaurant your school has. If you're lucky, the people who put food in your cafeteria will tell you the ingredients in the foods they serve. Which is pretty dang cool, because otherwise you might never know that the roasted red potatoes at Oregon State's Southside Station at Arnold are made with onion and garlic powder, just like the grilled chicken found in Harvard's salad bars. But you'll also be able to uncover the foods that suit your Go Low plan just fine, even if meals may wind up feeling a bit random and cobbled together. If your school doesn't list ingredients, you may be able to find contact information for a registered dietitian nutritionist who works with the school or the food-service company that provides food to your school. A friendly email to this person (refer to the script I gave you on page 100 for how to talk to a caf worker in person) can help you get to the bottom of things and assist you in finding a few go-to meals you can rely on.

# CHAPTER 6

## Nutrition Know-How

**N**utrition is a word you hear a lot, but there's much confusion about what good nutrition actually means. By definition, nutrition is "the act or process of nourishing or being nourished; the sum of the processes by which an animal or plant takes in and utilizes food substances." And while a FODMAP elimination and reintroduction may make sense for your specific health issue (like IBS), there's a lot more to eating well and nourishing your body than FODMAPs.

As a teenager, your body is growing—fast. Getting the nutrients you need is crucial for helping you be your best every day; it will also help set the stage for good health for the rest of your life. As much as 90 percent of your peak bone mass—how strong your bones are—will be formed by the time you're eighteen to twenty years old, for instance. That's *for life*—they don't get any stronger after that point. And that's just one example.

Because a low-FODMAP plan is by definition asking you to take a long list of foods out of your diet (at least temporarily), it is my responsibility as a registered dietitian nutritionist—and an all-around nice gal—to make sure you know how to restore the balance to your plate. In this chapter, I'll walk you through how to make sense of all the wacky nutrition information you hear out there, set you straight once and for all on which nutrients you need to eat, and clue you in on how to translate those details into food. We'll also talk about special concerns for vegetarians and vegans who want to Go Low and how to know if your efforts to "eat right" have gone too far. The good news: This insider information will help you stay healthy for years to come.

# NUTRITION FACTS: WHAT TO BELIEVE

Now, some days there seem to be as many opinions about nutrition as there are foods you can buy at your town's biggest grocery superstore. And you wouldn't be alone if you said that the vast amount of nutrition information that's out there—on *The Dr. Oz Show*, a recipe you found on a random blog, or what your friend was saying at lunch the other day—can be overwhelming, leaving you confused about what is real and what's not. Here's the thing about nutrition that many people miss: It's a science. Of course, science is about discoveries— and the people who study nutrition are constantly exploring and uncovering new information about how the way we eat affects our bodies. What's more, those "facts" are subject to interpretation—I've sat at a table listening to three registered dietitians discuss the same topic

and take the research to mean three completely different things. We're all interpreting what we learn all the time, even those of us who are "experts."

## Separating Nutrition Fact from Nutrition Fiction

So where does that leave you? Before we jump into our crash course on nutrition, I want to give you some tools to separate fact from fiction on your own.

*Look at the source:* Articles posted on government-sponsored websites and accounts (like choosemyplate.gov and letsmove.gov) are generally reputable, as are sites and streams run by trustworthy organizations like the Mayo Clinic (mayoclinic.org) or Cleveland Clinic (my.clevelandclinic.org/health). Sites run by commodity boards that represent the people who grow a specific type of food (like walnuts.org, run by the California Walnut Commission and Board) or a food brand (like clifbar.com) can be packed with great information but also exist for the purpose of promoting a product—so keep that in mind when you read them.

*Be mindful about blogs:* Some of the most widely read nutrition and health information out there these days comes from bloggers. And because anyone, I repeat, *anyone*, can have a blog, it's your job to decide whether the person is worth listening to. Does the blogger have a nutrition, medical, or other science-based degree from an accredited university (and not an online course or, worse, nothing)? Does he link to studies and/or other experts? Registered dietitians and registered dietitian nutritionists are often reputable sources of information because, by definition, they've passed a required set of courses focused on food and nutrition sciences; completed a supervised, roughly yearlong internship program working in various health care and food-service agencies; passed a certifying exam; and fulfilled requirements to keep up with continuing education credits and adhere to a professional code of ethics. Titles like "nutritionist" or "health counselor," however, might not mean much unless they're used in conjunction with a more established credential. So always be sure to dig a little deeper by clicking on your source's website and social media profiles to find out more about the background of the person providing the nutritional info.

*Reveal the research:* Reading up on nutrition? Studies and reports that have been reviewed by those in the same field of work (called peer-reviewed) and published in established journals are more worthy of your attention than a blog post written by Dr. Iknowitall, who also sells mysterious "miracle" supplements on her website. Now, it can be hard even for a person trained in nutrition to trudge through a journal article, and how to look for flaws in a study or cues that the research is solid is beyond what I can cover in the pages of this book. However, just knowing where to look is an excellent start. The website pubmed.gov is an invaluable resource for anyone interested in health and nutrition; it's a searchable, completely free database of biomedical and life sciences journal articles that's maintained by the National Institutes of Health's National Library of Medicine (NIH/NLM). If a nutrition topic shows up during your online travels, hit up PubMed to see what the scientific research is on the subject you're reading about—or if it even exists.

Let's say you read somewhere, "Eat fruit only on an empty stomach." Head over to PubMed and search the words "fruit," "empty," and "stomach." You'll pull up about twenty studies, none of which actually have anything to do with eating fruit on an empty stomach. If this claim was true, chances are you'd find something in the literature supporting it. Now, go ahead and search on PubMed for "FODMAP." Wow! You'll quickly see from the number of relevant articles that show up the difference between a well-researched nutrition topic and an Internet rumor.

*Be wary of absolutes and extremes:* "Gluten messes with your head!" "Coconut oil cures everything!" No doubt you've heard these dramatic claims or ones like them. But nutrition is far more nuanced than that. If someone says they have the answer to eating well—and it all comes down to eliminating one ingredient or entire food group, introducing one new magical superfood, or eating only something specific, like baby food, Twinkies, or meals at McDonald's (all "real diets"—google them!), chances are, it's too simple to be true.

*Red flag the cool, eye-catching graphics and the superhero treatment:* If you hear me screaming at my iPhone, it's probably because I'm losing my mind over all the comments, photos, and memes claiming expensive teas, shakes, and supplements are the secret to feeling and looking great. Or that perfectly-decent-but-not-magical ingredients (like turmeric) "melt body fat" or "chia seeds are the secret to long-lasting energy!" That's not to say

that behind every pretty picture is bad information. But when a claim goes only as deep as a flashy image, think twice about believing it.

Now that I've said all of that, I want to also make a case for keeping an open mind. Some diets that aren't well researched have helped people immensely. And on the other hand, some science-backed plans might just not cut it for your needs. Everyone is different, and you have every right to make the nutrition decisions that work best for you. However, I want you to do so in the most informed and balanced way possible. First rule: Don't make any big dietary decisions in a vacuum. If you're looking to make a major change in the way you eat, I strongly suggest that you work with a registered dietitian nutritionist who will help you—with an educated eye—sift through what's worth considering and what's bunk. My hope is that the next section of this book will help you become a better and more critical consumer of any nutrition-related information that crosses your path, digestive-health related or otherwise.

## HEALTHY EATING 101

When you think about why you eat, you may think *because I get hungry* or *because food tastes good.* And while those might both be true, the real reason we eat is to provide our bodies with fuel and other important compounds that help us survive. In fact, we have built-in mechanisms that cause us to get hungry and to derive pleasure from foods in order to encourage us to prioritize eating so we're more likely to stay healthy and strong.

Generally speaking, nutrients— components in food that help us survive and grow—come in two types: macronutrients and micronutrients. Macronutrients are those that provide our bodies with energy, like the gas you put in a car. Calories are the unit of measure we use to make sense of that energy. So when you look at two Nutrition Facts labels side by side and see that one food supplies 100 calories per serving and another 250 calories per serving, the 250-calorie food gives your body more energy to use. Sounds good enough, but the downside is that we live in a world where food is everywhere, and it's way too easy to get more energy or calories than you need each day. But we'll come back to that.

So, macronutrients, again, are the nutrients that give your body energy. Carbohydrates, which we've talked about quite a bit in this book because all FODMAPs are carbohydrates, are one type of macronutrient. They supply the body with 4 calories per gram. Protein— another type of macronutrient found in animal-based foods like chicken and eggs and certain plant foods like tofu and beans—also has 4 calories per gram. Fat—the third type of macronutrient—is found in foods like olive oil and butter and packs 9 calories per gram.

Going back to my car analogy, micronutrients are like the engine oil, windshield wiper fluid, and transmission fluid, which are super important for how well your vehicle works. Your car will turn on without them, but it may not run so smoothly. The equivalent of these in your body are the micronutrients known as vitamins and minerals. Your body needs them in small amounts—hence *micro*nutrients.

There's a long list of vitamins and minerals that are crucial for your body; you probably know far more of them than you think. The mineral calcium, for instance, is important for strong bones but also for how your muscles and nerves communicate. If your mom has ever tossed you zinc lozenges when you felt a cold coming on, that's because this mineral is linked with improved immunity, which is your body's ability to fight invaders. When you fall down and scrape your knee, vitamin K helps

## How Much Should I Weigh?

Having digestive troubles can take a toll on your overall well-being, as you know. For many people, frequent episodes of diarrhea can make it hard to stay at a healthy weight, or the fear of bringing on symptoms can result in decreased appetite or desire to eat (see page 125)—either or both of which can result in weight loss. And because digestive diseases look different depending on the person who has them, some people might actually gain weight, particularly if the foods that agree with them are high in calories but not very satisfying. So how do you know if the number you see on the scale is a healthy one? Body mass index, or BMI, is the best convenient method we have to assess body weight right now (there are more accurate methods, but they involve doing crazy things like getting weighed underwater or sitting in a futuristic "BOD POD"—seriously!). The BMI measure plots your height against your weight, which will tell you how you compare to other girls or guys your age. If you're younger than twenty, you'll want to look at your BMI-for-age on a growth chart. You can plug in the appropriate information on this website: nccd.cdc.gov/dnpabmi/calculator.aspx. If you're twenty or older, you'll use the adult BMI calculator here: cdc.gov/healthyweight/assessing/bmi/adult_bmi/english_bmi_calculator/bmi_calculator.html. Both sites will tell you whether your weight is considered healthy. If you're at either extreme, it would be helpful to meet with an RDN to help you reach your healthiest weight; the advice in this chapter will help you balance your diet, eat well, and build a healthier body.

your blood thicken and clot so you don't lose a pint; vitamin C helps the wound heal and form scar tissue (it's actually not as useful in fighting colds as people believe it to be). I could go on all day about all of the cool things different vitamins and minerals can do for you. . . .

But I won't. Because I haven't even mentioned antioxidants yet! (I know—does it get any cooler than my job?) If macronutrients are the gas and micronutrients are all the little helper fluids that keep a car running smoothly, antioxidants are the car washes that scrub your car down, shine it up, and vacuum out the inside. Antioxidants clean up the inside your body, preventing your cells from becoming damaged. Fruits and vegetables are the best sources of antioxidants, though other foods that come from plants, like beans, chocolate, and coffee, will also provide you with a hefty amount.

## HOW MANY CALORIES SHOULD I BE EATING?

All foods are some combination of one or more of the three macronutrients that provide your body with energy, or calories: carbohydrates, protein, and fats. If you've ever wondered how many calories you need, it's actually pretty easy to figure out. The number depends on a few factors like how old you are, whether you're a boy or girl, and how active you are. The easiest way to calculate your calorie needs is by visiting a website that does it for you; the USDA's Food and Nutrition Information Center has an easy-to-use one at fnic.nal.usda.gov/fnic/interactiveDRI. You can also download an app for your iPhone or Android; simply go to the app store and look for "USDA DRI Calculator for Healthcare Professionals" (I promise, you don't have to be a health care professional to use it).

If you want to do the math yourself, you can use the table on page 112 and your weight or height to figure it out. If you're at a healthy weight for your height and age, I'd use weight. If you're considered underweight or overweight, use height instead for a more relevant estimate. The first step is to translate your weight from pounds into kilograms, and your height from inches into centimeters. Google it, or use the equation below:

Pounds to kilograms = Pounds divided by 2.2

Inches to centimeters = Inches times 2.54 (in case you only know your height in feet, there are 12 inches per foot; so if you're 5 feet tall, you'd be 60 inches)

If you're a 100-pound, thirteen-year-old girl who falls into a healthy BMI range, you'd simply divide 100 pounds by 2.2 to get 45.5 kilograms. Multiply 45.5 kilograms by 47, and you'll see that you need roughly 2,138.5 calories per day.

## TYPES OF MACRONUTRIENTS

As for those macronutrients that provide your body with energy, each one is important to the body in many different

## CALORIE NEEDS

| AGE, BOYS | CALORIES PER KILOGRAM | CALORIES PER CENTIMETER |
|---|---|---|
| 11–14 | 55 | 15.9 |
| 15–18 | 45 | 17.1 |
| 19–24 | 40 | 16.4 |

| AGE, GIRLS | CALORIES PER KILOGRAM | CALORIES PER CENTIMETER |
|---|---|---|
| 11–14 | 47 | 14 |
| 15–18 | 40 | 13.5 |
| 19–24 | 38 | 13.4 |

ways. Here's what you need to know about them.

## Carbohydrates: Quality over Quantity

Carbohydrates get a bad rap, but they're so, so important. For starters, they're your brain's preferred source of energy. When researchers looked at the short-term effects of cutting carbs, women on such a diet were slower to react and had a harder time remembering things than those eating a moderate-carb diet. And while experts say that the brain may adapt to a low-carb diet over time, they're very concerned about the effect that cutting carbs may have on younger people, whose brains are still developing and growing.

What you need to think about when it comes to carbs is quality. Not all carbohydrates are created equal.

Take carb-containing foods like fruits, vegetables, beans, quinoa, and brown rice. Each one comes tied up in a neat little package with filling, blood-sugar-stabilizing fiber, as well as a range of important nutrients that provide your body with an array of health benefits. It drives me crazy—crazy!—when I hear people say they're not eating carbs, only to watch them down fruit-and-yogurt smoothies and giant bowls of salad. Fruits, vegetables, and yogurt are all made up of carbohydrates, albeit fewer carbohydrates than a big plate of pasta.

What people often actually mean when they say they're on a "low-carb diet" is that they're limiting the specific types of carbohydrates known as refined grains. A refined grain is one that has had some of its most beneficial parts removed—the nutritious parts known as the bran and the germ, which also contain fiber that helps fill you up and regulate your digestive tract. What's left is the inside part, known as the endosperm, which contains the starch, or sugar, that provides the body (and plant) with energy. When you eat a whole-grain food like brown rice, the germ and the bran work with the endosperm to slow down the rate at which your body breaks down the starch and delivers it to your cells. So in general, anything made with whole wheat flour wins over just plain old wheat flour (also called all-purpose flour)—bread, pasta, flour tortillas, muffins, cookies, and more. Easy, you're thinking—wheat is high FODMAP, so I'm not going to be eating too much of it anyway. Wheat, however, is not the only grain that gets refined. White rice, as well as anything made with white rice flour or cornstarch (as many gluten-free products are), is also considered a refined grain.

Grain foods (refined or not) are considered complex carbohydrates. This means they are made up primarily of long chains of sugar molecules—the building blocks of all carbohydrates. Smaller sugars are referred to as *simple sugars*—and with these, quality counts, too.

You've probably figured out by now that sugar isn't just the white stuff your grandma pours into her famous chocolate chip cookies (technically, that's called sucrose, or table sugar). Simple sugars occur naturally in foods like fruits and milk; those aren't the ones you need to worry about. Added sugars, such as those in table sugar, high-fructose corn syrup, brown sugar, and even in sweeteners perceived as more "natural," like honey and maple syrup, add carbohydrates to your diet without any dietary bonuses like significant amounts of vitamins, minerals or fiber, not to mention they're easy to consume in excess.

Wondering what carbohydrate-predominant foods will fit into a Go Low plan? As long as you stick with proper portion sizes (see page 57), you can try any of the following.

### GRAINS

(choose the less-refined, higher fiber ones as often as possible)

- Go Low–approved gluten-free versions of bread, cereal, pasta, and baking mix (used to make muffins, pancakes, etc.) as well as oats/oatmeal, quinoa, buckwheat, potato, white rice, brown rice, sorghum

### PRODUCE

- Arugula, banana, bell peppers, blueberries, bok choy, cantaloupe, carrots, celery, eggplant, grapes, honeydew, kale, lettuce, parsnips, pineapple, potatoes, spinach, strawberries, yellow squash, zucchini

**SWEETENERS**
(use conservatively to avoid excess calories)
- Maple syrup, granulated sugar, brown sugar

## Protein Power!

Protein is having a moment in the spotlight like a YouTube video gone viral, and let's let it have that—protein is undoubtedly an important part of our diets. Every cell in your body contains protein, after all. Getting protein in your diet ensures that your body can build and repair muscles, bones, and skin, and even make new hair; it's also valuable for helping curb your appetite, because people feel more satisfied after protein-rich meals than they do carbohydrate-heavy ones.

So there's no doubt that protein plays a crucial role in our well-being; the question for many people, however, is "How much protein do I need?" Here's where I may clash with people pushing protein powders or a Paleo-style diet—my answer is "Probably not as much

as you think." The recommended protein intake for a teenager is 40 to 60 grams per day, although the specifics depend on factors like your size and gender. A study that reviewed data from a large national health survey called the National Health and Nutrition Examination Survey found that most people were getting enough protein each day. The researchers did notice, however, that 7.7 percent of teenage girls reported getting less than the recommended amount—teen boys didn't seem to have the same problem. Chances are you're getting enough protein; however, it's not a bad idea to take some time to make sure you're on target.

To estimate how much you need, you'll have to do a little math. It's simple, I promise. Again, you can use either your weight or height to figure it out—if you're at a healthy weight for your height and age, go ahead and use weight; if you're considered to be in the underweight or overweight range, use height instead for a more useful estimate. The first step, again, is to translate your weight from pounds into kilograms, and your height from inches into centimeters. Google it, or use this equation:

## PROTEIN NEEDS

| AGE, BOYS | GRAMS PER KILOGRAM | GRAMS PER CENTIMETER |
|-----------|--------------------|----------------------|
| 11–14 | 1.0 | 0.29 |
| 15–18 | 0.9 | 0.34 |
| 19–24 | 0.8 | 0.33 |

| AGE, GIRLS | GRAMS PER KILOGRAM | GRAMS PER CENTIMETER |
|------------|--------------------|----------------------|
| 11–14 | 1.0 | 0.29 |
| 15–18 | 0.8 | 0.27 |
| 19–24 | 0.8 | 0.28 |

Pounds to kilograms = Pounds divided by 2.2

Inches to centimeters = Inches times 2.54 (in case you only know your height in feet, there are 12 inches per foot; so if you're 5 feet tall, you'd be 60 inches)

If you're a 100-pound, thirteen-year-old girl who falls into a healthy BMI range, you'd simply divide 100 pounds by 2.2 to get 45.5 kilograms. Multiply 45.5 kilograms by 1, and you'll see that you need roughly 45.5 grams of protein per day.

Here are some protein-predominant foods that will fit nicely into your Go Low plan. Just make sure to stay within the recommended portion sizes given in Chapter 4.

**MEATS**
- Any type, including chicken, turkey, beef, pork, and bacon (just be mindful of seasonings and marinades)

**FISH**
- Any type, including salmon, tuna, flounder, tilapia, and cod

**PLANT-BASED PROTEIN**
- Firm tofu; tempeh; nuts like macadamia, brazil, peanuts, and pecans; seeds like chia, pumpkin, sesame, and sunflower (seeds and nuts are considered sources of both protein and fat); small servings of canned lentils and chickpeas (see page 122 for more on vegetarian FODMAPs)

**OTHER**
- Eggs, hard cheeses

## What About Protein Powder?

As a registered dietitian nutritionist who also happens to have been a vegetarian since age twelve, I always have people asking me what kind of protein powder I like. They're usually surprised when I say none. Most people I work with—particularly teenagers—do just fine in the protein department without any powdered supplements. I find that people do best on a low-FODMAP plan when they're able to strip their diet down to the basics. And because protein powders usually have long lists of ingredients (often off-limits sweeteners or the digestive disruptors inulin or chicory root), you're introducing a lot of room for high-FODMAP complications. If you plan on ignoring my advice, powders sourced from rice protein, egg protein, and whey protein are considered low FODMAP—talk to a registered dietitian nutritionist who can help you find one to best meet your needs. However, keep in mind that Go Low–approved foods like lactose-free yogurt, lactose-free kefir, and peanut butter all add a lower-risk protein punch. You can also try a new low-FODMAP-approved meal replacement shake by Nestlé called ProNourish Low FODMAP Nutritional Drink, which packs 15 grams of protein per serving (check ingredients to decide if it's right for you).

## Phat Fats

People have been fearful of fat—another misunderstood nutrient—for decades. This probably goes back to 1980, when the government released a set of dietary guidelines that advised people to reduce the amount of fat in their diets. As a result, companies began inventing products to feed this "fat phobia"—nonfat salad dressings, low-fat cheeses, and even fat-free cookies—and people ate more carbohydrates (usually the sugary and refined ones) as a result.

We know now that fat is not to be feared—the most recent version of the *Dietary Guidelines for Americans* even dropped the fat restriction for the first time since 1980. In addition to providing energy, fat helps your body absorb vitamins A, D, E, and K— otherwise known as the fat-soluble vitamins. In other words, if you eat that salad with vinegar and no oil, your body won't be able to use many of the valuable vitamins in the veggies. Fats are important parts of healthy cell membranes, make hormones, help your hair shine and your skin glow, and much more.

Different types of fat, however, can have different impacts on your body. The omega-3 fats found in fish (a mainly protein food) like salmon, tuna, and sardines; walnuts and walnut oil; and flaxseed and flax oil can help reduce the risk of heart disease. Monounsaturated fats are linked with decreasing bad LDL cholesterol and are found in nuts like walnuts, macadamias, and pecans; in oils like sunflower, canola, and avocado; and in fruits we think of as vegetables, like avocados and olives.

On the other end of the spectrum are man-made trans fats that are created when manufacturers turn liquid oil into a solid form. Food companies frequently used these fats in packaged foods because they helped stabilize products to give them a longer shelf life. According to the Institute of Medicine, there is no known safe level of consumption of trans fats, because they increase the level of bad LDL cholesterol while decreasing the level of good HDL cholesterol—a double whammy for heart health. They also increase inflammation, which is at the core of many diseases like diabetes and heart disease. The food industry has since cut the amount of trans fats in many foods, and the Food and Drug Administration is taking steps to have them removed from processed foods. You may still, however, find them lurking in some. It's also worth noting that a small amount of naturally occurring trans fats are present in some meat and dairy foods; however, researchers are not sure if they have the same impact as the man-made ones.

Somewhere in the middle are saturated fats. Years ago, you would have heard that saturated fats are all bad—linked with increases in cholesterol and heart disease risk—but we're now learning that saturated fats may be a bit more complicated than that. The saturated fats found in animal foods like meat and dairy seem most likely to increase cholesterol, while those in plant foods like coconut oil and chocolate might not have any impact. What's more, there may be a difference between the compositions of fat in beef from a grain-fed cow that's spent time in a feedlot, compared with that from a grass-fed cow that was raised on a farm. When it comes to saturated fats, the most important point to keep in mind might be what you could be eating instead. If you cut saturated fats only to eat more refined carbs, you might increase your risk for heart disease. Swap saturated fats with polyunsaturated ones like those in nuts and fish? You'll likely be helping your heart.

There's no reason to be afraid of fat, particularly the beneficial plant- and fish-based kinds. Here are the fat-predominant foods you can have in the proper proportions (see pages 55 to 59) when you're Going Low.

### OILS
- Olive oil, canola oil, sunflower oil, flax oil, avocado oil, walnut oil, garlic-infused olive oil.

### NUTS AND SEEDS
(also a good sources of protein)
- Chia seeds, sesame seeds, sunflower seeds, macadamia nuts, pecans, pine nuts, walnuts, peanuts, peanut butter

### VEGETABLES
- ⅛ avocado, olives

## SO WHAT AM I SUPPOSED TO EAT, AGAIN?

Now that you know all about the nutrients that are important to your body, you know what to eat, right? Of course not! The detail that many people miss when talking about nutrition is

that we don't eat grams of protein or carbohydrates. We eat food. And while the purpose of eating food is to supply your body with crucial energy, vitamins, minerals, and antioxidants, if we don't discuss it in terms of actual food, you're really not going to care too much. So let's shift gears and talk about how to put all of this nutrition information on your plate.

Well, MyPlate!

## Building Meals with MyPlate

In 2011, the US Department of Agriculture introduced MyPlate (choosemyplate.gov), a tool designed to help people figure out how to eat. Funnily enough, I was already using a similar graphic in my nutrition counseling practice to teach people how to build a healthy meal. So I was thrilled to see the plate concept grow in popularity. Here's the gist of it. You eat a meal off a plate—sure, sometimes you eat from a bowl or a bag while you're running down the hall to get to your next class. But in general, you can easily envision what a meal on a plate looks like. Your goal:

**1.** Fill one half of the plate with produce.

# Going Coco-nuts?

I'm not sure what it is about coconuts, but it seems everyone is nuts for coconut oil and other coconutty ingredients lately. Good news: This fat is carbohydrate-free and therefore low in FODMAPs (serving size: 1 tablespoon). Experts say that it's not quite as bad for your blood cholesterol as butter, but it can still have a negative impact. On the positive side, though, it may have some antimicrobial benefits, among others. I recommend using virgin coconut oil in moderation; its nutty and slightly sweet flavor is perfect for roasting vegetables and sautéing greens. It also makes a suitable dairy-free butter substitute for baking. Oh, but don't go too coconut crazy— coconut water is high in FODMAPs, and dried coconut is only OK in no more than ¼ cup (20 g) servings. Coconut milk from a can (the thick kind that you'd use in a recipe) is OK in up to ½ cup (120 ml) amounts; refrigerated coconut milk that you'd put in your cereal hasn't yet been tested for its FODMAP content.

**2.** Fill one quarter with protein.

**3.** Fill one quarter with grains (preferably whole grains).

That's it! The plate doesn't give a separate section for fat, because you'll likely ingest the small amount you need each day through fats like oil used to cook or dress your meal, or nuts and avocado on a salad, without thinking too much about it.

I love how simple this concept is and how easily you can apply it to your next meal—and every time you eat, for that matter. Let's walk through it a couple of times so you can see how easy it is to put a meal on MyPlate.

## MyPlate and Low FODMAPs

Imagine you're at a bagel brunch with a table full of toppings and assorted breakfast items. Your instinct (if you're not Going Low, of course) could be to select a bagel with butter. As you know from the first part of this chapter, that would give you a whole lot of those not-so-great refined carbohydrates and some fat—not exactly the picture of that balanced plate you're striving for.

Instead, you could take just half a whole wheat bagel, top it with smoked salmon, egg salad, or peanut butter for protein, and have some chopped cucumber and tomato or fruit salad for your produce on the side. Voilà—a MyPlate meal.

Now think of a typical Go Low scenario. You need an easy breakfast and notice that EnviroKidz Gorilla Munch is one of the cereals that is Go Low approved. Great! So you put some in a bag and munch on it while you're on the bus to school. *Screeeeeeech* (that's the sound of the school bus braking so you can run back home and put that breakfast on MyPlate)! OK. You have your grains. So what's missing? You've got it, protein and produce. Toss a single-serving lactose-free yogurt into your bag along with a medium banana. Now you're good to go.

It's important to remember the principles of MyPlate as you're working through the various stages of the Go Low plan. With the world of restrictions you open up when you go low FODMAP, it can be easy to toss overall diet quality out the window and simply focus on, well, finding the first food you can eat without having any trouble (as in the Gorilla Munch–in-a-baggie scenario I laid out earlier). And that's totally understandable. But the little bit of extra effort you put into balancing out your meals and snacks will make your food not only more nutritious but also more interesting to eat and more satisfying. In other words, it will help you stick with it for long enough to feel better, reintroduce foods, and arrive at a happy place for your belly that you can keep up for good.

## COMMON FODMAP MISTAKES

Following a low-FODMAP plan can cause you to fall into some not-so-good nutrition traps, so while you're helping one problem, you might be creating another. Here are a few frequently seen FODMAPer don'ts.

### Don't Pile on the Protein

If you're a low FODMAPer who loves meat, fish, and eggs, that's fine. These foods are FODMAP-free because they don't contain any carbohydrates, and safe for you to eat. You don't, however, want to overdo them. Too much protein can make your kidneys work harder than they need to; it can also weaken your bones. Eating large amounts of red meat, in particular, as a teen is associated with a greater risk of developing breast cancer as an adult, according to a study of women published in the *International*

*Journal of Cancer.* And eating an excess of protein from animal foods may also cause problems in the gut. The fermentation that occurs in the colon as a result can produce potentially hazardous compounds. Researchers are beginning to explore the role this might play in gut disorders.

## Don't Forget the Fiber

It's not uncommon for low FODMAPers to shy away from foods like whole grains and vegetables that can, in excess, cause digestive distress. But by doing so, you may be unintentionally decreasing your intake of fiber, a compound in food that under normal circumstances helps add bulk to your stools and keep material moving through your digestive tract (it also helps regulate water content in poop). If you are already eating a low-fiber diet, it's better to gradually increase the amount you're eating—but the portion-size restrictions on the Go Low plan should help keep you from going too fast too soon.

## Don't Fear Fruit

It can be intimidating to look at the list of foods you can eat on the Go Low plan and realize that healthy items you've never thought twice about eating—like apples, pears, mangos, and cherries—

may be giving you digestive problems. But don't drop the fruit from your diet so fast! The ones you *can* eat—like bananas, blueberries, and strawberries—can give you more of that all-important fiber, vitamins like wound-healing vitamin C, minerals like blood-pressure-lowering potassium, and disease-fighting antioxidants—not to mention a pop of sweet, fresh flavor. Just keep your fruit intake to no more than one serving per meal or snack.

## Don't Skip Snacks

If you normally munch on a high-FODMAP food like crackers or applesauce when you get home from school, you might be inclined to just wait until dinner to eat. But going long stretches of time without eating can leave you tired and hangry (hungry-angry). It can also set you up for failure later in the day—the hungrier you get, the more likely you are to grab the first food you see, low FODMAP or not. The good news: There are plenty of low-FODMAP snacks to choose from; see page 64 for ideas.

## Don't Overdo Oils

Because fat-only or primarily fat foods like olive oil and mayonnaise contain no FODMAPs, some low FODMAPers see that as a green light to eat as much as they'd like. Eating too much fat, however, can also cause digestive upset. Enjoy a little bit of olive oil drizzled onto your salad or on top of your gluten-free bread, and definitely put some mayo on those turkey lettuce wraps. Just don't go crazy.

## Don't Let Perfection Stand in the Way of Progress

There is no such thing as a perfect diet. And whether your diet has restrictions or not, sometimes doing your best is the best you can do—and that's good enough. Don't stress if you can't find a low-FODMAP fruit or vegetable to round out your meal or if you're at a rest stop and the only acceptable snack available is a bag of tortilla chips. Nutrition is all about balance, and if you're regularly making choices that move you toward a healthier diet—all with the added challenge of finding the foods that don't irritate your gut—step back and look at the big picture. You're probably doing great! And if the panoramic view's not so hot? Your next meal—a.k.a. your next opportunity to do your best—is right around the corner.

# SPECIAL NUTRITION CONCERNS

Each person who attempts a low-FODMAP plan has a different low-FODMAP experience. If you already follow a limited diet like a vegetarian or vegan one, there are certain things you need to know about Going Low. And everyone who considers a low-FODMAP plan should be aware of how dietary restriction can affect your relationship with food and your body.

## Vegetarian and Vegan FODMAPers

If you're someone who doesn't eat meat (like me, since age twelve!), a low-FODMAP plan can feel even more overwhelming. The main reason: Much of the food that helps keep a vegetarian diet well balanced is high in FODMAPs. For instance, beans like kidney beans and black beans (not to mention canned lentils in amounts larger than ½ cup/ 45 g per serving and canned chickpeas in amounts larger than ¼ cup/40 g per serving), silken tofu, cashews, almond butter, hummus, edamame, and soy milk can all be problematic. And if you're a vegan—a person who consumes no animal products whatsoever—you're already more limited because the cheeses, lactose-free yogurt, and eggs a lacto-ovo vegetarian (a person who eats no meat but does consume dairy and eggs) might eat for protein are off your plate. But trust me, because I've been there—being a vegetarian or vegan while you Go Low is completely doable. Here are a few strategies for low FODMAPers to keep in mind:

*Make it short and sweet:* Because your diet will be rather limited, particularly for vegans, you'll want to keep your Go Low elimination phase as short as possible. If you feel relief after a few days, as many low FODMAPers do, start phase two (reintroduction) at two weeks. If at two weeks in you're still not feeling great, fine-tune your Go Low plan just a bit and give it another week.

*End your dependence on beans— for now:* The biggest challenge of Going Low for many vegetarians is the restriction on legumes like beans, peas, and more. The good news is that you can eat chickpeas and lentils in very small amounts and specific circumstances. The first catch: They must be canned, drained, and rinsed well; all of that time sitting in water actually helps leach some FODMAPs from the beans. The second: You can have only a small amount—up to ½ cup (45 g) canned lentils and up to ¼ cup (40 g) canned chickpeas.

*Don't shy away from soy:* Soybeans themselves (also known as edamame in Japanese restaurants) are high in FODMAPs, as is soy milk (technically it depends on how the soy milk is made, but to be safe, assume it's all off-limits). However, depending on how the soybeans are processed, they may be OK. Tofu is a low-FODMAP food, as long as you stick with the firm and extra firm varieties, as they've had many of the offending carbohydrates drained off. You can also press your firm tofu to make it even lower in FODMAPs: Place a block of tofu on a plate covered with a few paper towels, top with a few more paper towels and a cutting board or plate and a heavy item like a book or pot. Allow it to sit for thirty to sixty minutes, and discard any liquid that appears. Avoid silken tofu, which is a no-no. Tempeh should be OK, though I've seen clients have trouble with it. If you suspect you have trouble tolerating it, skip it during phase one and try reintroducing it later on.

*Get to know nuts and seeds:* You do have to watch serving sizes, but nuts and seeds like peanuts (and peanut butter), sunflower seeds, pumpkin seeds, chia seeds, walnuts, Brazil nuts, and macadamia nuts are all good sources of protein.

*Choose your grains wisely:* Some grains are better sources of protein than others. Grains like quinoa, buckwheat, amaranth, teff, and sorghum in approved serving sizes are all smart picks.

## Plant-Powered Go Low Proteins

If you're vegetarian or vegan, these are the foods you can safely use to bump up your protein intake:

- Firm or extra firm tofu

- Tempeh

- Seitan

- Nuts: walnuts, macadamias, Brazil, pecans, peanuts, peanut butter

- Seeds: pumpkin, sesame, chia, sunflower

- Grains: quinoa, amaranth, teff, buckwheat, sorghum

- Canned lentils

- Canned chickpeas

*Try some meat alternatives:* Have you ever had mock duck or fake chicken in a Chinese restaurant? If so, it was probably made from seitan (*SAY-tan*). Seitan is an alternative meat product made from the protein found in wheat, called wheat gluten. Sound familiar? That's because it's exactly what people with celiac disease and those who are gluten sensitive cannot eat. For low FODMAPers who can tolerate gluten, however, seitan is thought to be a suitable choice (remember, low FODMAP is all about carbohydrates—so even though wheat is not OK, wheat gluten can be because it's the protein separated from the fermentable carbs).

And one more thing, my vegetarian friend. Pretty much all of the recipes at the end of this book are vegetarian, or easily vegetarian adaptable in addition to being low FODMAP and gluten-free. A bunch are even vegan. I hope you love them all!

## Gut Disorders and Disordered Eating

It's easy to understand how issues with your stomach could affect your relationship with food. Living in fear that eating will make you feel terrible or embarrass yourself is enough to make anyone feel negative about food. And when you realize that limiting what

# When Your Gut Gets in the Way of Life

Problems with digestive health, as you likely know, can take a real toll on your overall well-being. In addition the potential overlap with eating disorders, having gut problems has been linked with other mental health issues as well. In some cases, researchers don't always know which issue causes which—or if they coexist and feed off one another. However, here are some conditions you may be at an increased risk for if you're living with a gastrointestinal illness. As in the case of disordered eating, speak with a health professional immediately if any of these sound like you.

**DEPRESSION:** Adults with symptoms of functional gut disorders—whether or not they'd been formally diagnosed by their doctor—were twice as likely to exhibit signs of depression or anxiety, according to a study done at two hospitals in Ontario, Canada; it seems that younger people are no different, say experts. And as many as 20 to 40 percent of teens with IBD have depressive symptoms, according to a study published in the journal *BMJ Open Gastroenterology* that looked at how to effectively treat these disorders.

**ANXIETY:** Roughly half of people with IBS surveyed by researchers in Poland had experienced clinical anxiety at some point in their lives—symptoms ranging from social phobias to generalized anxiety disorder to agoraphobia (fear of certain places and situations). And people with Crohn's and colitis are twice as likely to experience generalized anxiety disorder at some point in their lives, compared with people who do not have IBD, according to a study from Canada. Women, say researchers, were four times as likely to be affected as men.

**OPIOID ABUSE:** People younger than the age of eighteen with IBD are more likely than their healthy peers to overuse prescription painkillers, according to a study from the University of North Carolina. Those with depression and/or anxiety were even more likely to overdo the pills.

**SUICIDE:** Scary but true—people with IBD have higher rates of suicide than their healthy peers. And the same may be true for people with IBS—one study found that 38 percent of IBS patients who sought the care of specialists at one UK medical center had contemplated suicide because of their symptoms. If suicide is a thought that

*continues* ➜

crosses your mind, seek help immediately. The National Suicide Prevention Lifeline is 800-273-8255, and it's open 24 hours a day, 7 days a week. And remember that doctors, school counselors, and more are always available to talk. You are not alone.

GI issues can make you feel helpless and lost, nervous and desperate. But help and support are available from friends, family, your health care team, and perfect strangers, if you take the initiative to find it. I urge you to take the initiative today if you are in need. This, too, shall pass.

you eat can improve your symptoms, it can encourage you to try to feel even more empowered by limiting what you eat more than necessary. What's more, the relationship between eating disorders and digestive problems might work the other way around—meaning, people who have eating disorders may be negatively affecting their digestive health as well. Here's what you need to know about the intersection of gut disorders and eating disorders.

**Know you're at risk:** There's a clear correlation between people with eating disorders and those with gut problems: Roughly 98 percent of 101 female patients admitted to an eating disorder unit at a hospital in Australia fit the criteria for functional gut disorders; half specifically met the criteria for IBS.

Researchers aren't exactly sure if it's the gut disorder that causes the eating disorder or the other way around—but either way, as a person with GI issues, it's important to know that the two can have quite a bit of overlap, and be aware of any signs your relationship with food has gone bad.

**Recognize the signs:** Are you restricting the food you're eating beyond the parameters of the low-FODMAP or another diet you may be on as recommended by your doctor or registered dietitian nutritionist? Do you binge or purge or use laxatives or diuretics? Are your eating patterns erratic? Do you alter your schedule so you can conveniently skip meals or eating occasions? Do you feel strong shame or guilt about your eating habits?

Keep in mind that behaviors and emotions that may not exactly meet the definition of anorexia, bulimia, or binge eating may still be classified as an eating disorder not otherwise specified (EDNOS) or simply disordered eating—and any of the above deserve special attention.

Talk to someone: Having a digestive illness is a good enough reason to regularly meet with a psychologist, social worker, school counselor, or someone else whom you can speak with openly about your challenges, concerns, and fears. But if you have a gut disorder coupled with any disordered eating behavior, the need is even greater. Ask your doctor, registered dietitian nutritionist, or school nurse for a referral; if for some reason you cannot find someone to talk to in person, you can also try the National Eating Disorders Association helpline at 800-931-2237; check out their website at nationaleatingdisorders.org, where you'll also find an online chat helpline, an eating disorders screening quiz, and more valuable resources.

Reverse "food is the enemy" thinking: It may be true that eating certain things sends your digestive health into a tailspin. However, the right foods are also nourishment, energy, and healing. If you've long gotten anxious around mealtimes, it can be hard to turn this thinking around—part of the reason talking with a trained professional is crucial. But uncovering the foods that make you feel well and strong as you learn to manage the ones that give you problems, as you've been doing throughout the course of your low-FODMAP plan, is a huge step you can take in your journey to rebuild your relationship with food. Focus on those foods and how you feel when you eat them. And with the help of a trained therapist, do everything you can to change that dialogue in your head.

# CHAPTER 7

## Balancing Belly Bugs:
### YOUR MICROBIOME, PROBIOTICS, AND MORE

D o you ever get that funny feeling that you're not alone? Because it turns out, you're really not, and you never have been. Inside your GI tract are tens of trillions of teeny tiny bugs, also known as microorganisms. This is less creepy than it sounds, I promise, because it's completely normal— actually, it's essential to human life. Everyone has a different combination of these little invisible critters inhabiting them—a delicate ecosystem known as your *microbiome*.

As you know by now, your microbiome has a lot to do with your gut health, among other aspects of your well-being. If you have IBS, the symptoms you experience (diarrhea, constipation, or both) might be linked with the kinds of microorganisms in your digestive tract. And the more researchers learn about links between genetics and the microbiomes of people with inflammatory bowel diseases, the closer they get to developing effective strategies to prevent and treat them.

Your microbiome starts developing the second you are born, and will look different depending on whether you were a cesarean or vaginal birth, whether you were breast- or bottle-fed, and even what was in the air and who held you at the hospital. From there, your microbiome evolves, becoming more and more personalized based on factors such as what you eat, your stress level, and how often you take antibiotics for something like strep throat or an ear infection (antibiotics kill the bad bacteria that make you sick, but they also zap some good bacteria along the way). Each person's microbiome is a microscopic fingerprint, something that is completely unique to him or her—but unlike a fingerprint that stays the same your whole life, your microbiome is always changing.

In addition to gut health, research links the makeup of your microbiome with everything from how well your immune system fights off viruses to your emotional well-being to your weight (in some cases, researchers aren't sure if it's the chicken or the egg—in other words, does a microbiome that looks a certain way cause a person to feel happier, or does a person who feels happier have a microbiome that looks a certain way?). It's fascinating stuff, and the research—like your microbiome—is constantly evolving.

As for those bugs: Chances are you grew up believing that *bacteria* was a bad word, and *yeast* was something bakers used to make bread rise, am I right? So it might surprise you to learn that certain types of bacteria and yeasts can also serve and help your body. Probiotics are good microorganisms (bacteria and yeasts) that can help destroy disease-causing bugs, boost your immune system, and more.

Probiotics sound like an easy solution to some complicated problems. If good gut health is linked with certain patterns in the microbiome, why not just give people more of the probiotic strains (a.k.a. types) they need? Won't that help get belly problems sorted out? Unfortunately, it's not that simple— because as far as your gut is concerned, it's not just about getting more probiotics. The magic word in digestion is *balance*.

## Dysbiosis Defined

*Dysbiosis* is a word you may hear at a doctor's office or read about on health blogs that refers to an imbalance of microbes. In other words, there are too many not-so-good bugs and not enough of the beneficial guys.

Eating well is one important part of striking that balance. And it's not just about being on a special gut-health diet (sticking with a low-FODMAP plan for too long can actually hurt you; see page 91 for details)—when scientists look at mice eating a so-called Western diet—in other words, the processed foods that are high in fat and sugar that many people in the United States eat regularly—they find an overgrowth of bad bugs that increase inflammation, like E. coli, and a decrease in protective bacteria. And fiber, it seems, is a crucial component of eating right for your microbiome—getting plenty ensures that the good bugs in your gut have plenty of food to munch on, which helps them thrive and protects the lining of your gut, decreasing your risk of infection. So eating a diet that is generally healthy and fiber-rich is crucial.

## TRYING PROBIOTICS

Adding in probiotic supplements (they come in the form of pills and powders and sometimes even chewables) is another strategy you can try to help balance out that gut. While many experts agree that probiotics in the diet are generally a good thing, there is a lot of confusion about which probiotics to recommend to whom and how to use them. What follows is a plan you can follow to find the probiotics that are right for you.

### Step One: Do Your Homework

The research on probiotics is growing, so do some research to find out the latest science. I've provided some of the probiotic brands and strains that have the most research behind them (as of this writing) that you're most likely to hear about and whom they might help (there are loads on the market, however, so this is only a small sampling):

**Culturelle (*Lactobacillus* GG):** Research links taking this probiotic with a decrease in pain and other symptoms in kids with the various forms of IBS; however, some of the products in the Culturelle line do contain inulin, which is high in FODMAPs—so only the inulin-free versions like Culturelle Health & Wellness are appropriate for anyone on the Go Low plan.

**Align (*Bifidobacterium infantis*):** When scientists looked at this probiotic, they found that it decreased inflammation in the intestines and can reduce symptoms of IBS. It may be a good choice for a person with diarrhea-predominant IBS or alternating diarrhea and constipation.

VSL#3: This very potent supplement is a mix of eight different probiotic strains, including several different types of lactobacilli and bifidobacteria. Research finds that it might help reduce symptoms in people with ulcerative colitis, pouchitis (an inflammation of the man-made rectum that a person might have if he's had surgery to remove a diseased colon), and constipation-predominant IBS (at a lower dose than someone with the other conditions).

*Bifidobacterium lactis:* This is a strain of probiotic that's currently found in some blends; several studies have found it to help move things along for people with constipation-predominant IBS. Double-check to make sure that any product you buy containing *Bifidobacterium lactis* doesn't contain a No ingredient.

## Step Two: Talk to Your Doctor or Registered Dietitian Nutritionist

Depending on your diagnosis, your doctor or dietitian may have specific recommendations—or suggest skipping the probiotics altogether (if that's the case, be sure to ask about whether you should eat fermented foods, as discussed later in this chapter).

## Step Three: Be Consistent

You won't know if the probiotic is working for you if you forget to take it half the time. Choose one time each day when you're most likely to remember to take your probiotic supplement—maybe pour the powder into your morning smoothie (if you do a blended drink each day, that is) or take it every night when you brush your teeth. Tying the action of taking a pill every day to something you already do daily without thinking about it too much is an effective way to create a new habit.

## Step Four: Give It a Month

Digestive health pros say that this is an adequate length of time to determine whether a probiotic is helping you. If after a month you feel it's not working, you can discontinue it. Go back to steps one and two and consider other probiotics you might try or save your money and stick with other tools. And if at any point you find that the probiotic is making your symptoms worse, drop it—stat.

# BUGS WITH YOUR BREAKFAST?

Pills and powders aren't the only places you can get probiotics from. These beneficial bugs occur naturally in fermented foods. Fermentation is a process by which microorganisms transform a food into another product. Before you think, "Hey, that sounds weird," you should know that you've undoubtedly eaten fermented foods throughout your life. Everyday foods like yogurt, sauerkraut, pickles, some cottage cheeses, and sourdough bread are produced through the process of fermentation. And less common to the United States—but growing in popularity—are fermented foods like kefir, kombucha, Korean kimchi, and even some foods that don't begin with *K*, like tempeh and miso.

Before we had factories that could produce shelf-stable cans and jars for storing vegetables (and more) over the long term, fermentation was used in many cultures as a way of preserving foods. And interestingly enough, these practices have been associated with good health for generations. Unfortunately, the most convincing research on probiotics has been done on supplements. However, it stands to reason that including fermented foods in your everyday diet is a wise decision for your gut and your overall health. Added bonus: Fermenting certain foods might actually break down their FODMAPs (a.k.a. the carbohydrates likely to give you a problem) and make them OK to eat even when you're on Go Low. Here are some ways you can include fermented foods in a low-FODMAP plan.

## Yogurt

Phase one of the Go Low plan includes lactose-free yogurt, preferably in plain flavor. Why plain? It limits the possibility of unwanted ingredients that might upset your gut. Many people can also tolerate strained yogurts like Greek yogurt and its Icelandic cousin, *skyr*. If you do OK with lactose-free yogurt and are ready to start reintroducing foods, you may want to experiment with small amounts of these yogurts (unsweetened as well); start with a couple of tablespoons at a time and work your way up to a typical serving.

Look for: Plain, lactose-free yogurt (phase one). Experiment with plain, regular strained varieties (like Greek or skyr) in phase two.

Use it: Mixed into Belly Balancing Overnight Oats (page 153); in individual serving cups as an easy on-the-go snack or light breakfast

## Kefir

Phase one of the Go Low plan also includes lactose-free kefir. Once you're on to phase two, you can also experiment with plain (unsweetened) kefir that is not lactose-free. The reason? The process of fermenting kefir actually cuts down on the lactose significantly. One brand to look for is Lifeway Kefir—the company claims its kefir is 99 percent lactose-free due to a long fermentation time.

## Sauerkraut

While many low-FODMAP blogs routinely include sauerkraut in recipes, my understanding is that sauerkraut is approved only in small amounts—1 tablespoon at a time. I recommend being cautious and holding off on kraut until you're in phase two, then introducing it as you would any other

## MAKING YOUR WAY IN THE KITCHEN

"I have learned a lot about cooking . . . and how strong I am."

"Try new foods so you have more options!"

"Cooking for myself helps me eat super clean."

"At first I ate hardly anything, but then I found that there are so many low-FODMAP recipes online. Now I prepare those so I get enough calories."

food—for three consecutive days, starting with a small amount (1 tablespoon). Later you can try to work your way up to a typical, moderate serving (no more than ¼ cup/80 g).

**Look for:** Refrigerated sauerkrauts made with cabbage, salt, and not much more. The ones on the shelf have been pasteurized, which kills the beneficial microbes.

**Use it:** As a topping on a Go Low–friendly rice bowl or salad

### Tempeh

Tempeh—made from fermented soybeans—is one example of a food that begins its life high in FODMAPs but becomes lower in FODMAPs once it's been fermented. Tempeh has a nutty, grainy texture similar to that of a veggie burger. It's also a great source of plant-based protein, perfect for Go Low vegetarians who can tolerate it (while it does test low for FODMAPs, some people still seem to have a problem digesting it; this is one food to add into your diet slowly). Up to around 3.5 ounces (100 g) is considered low FODMAP.

**Look for:** Plain tempeh—seasoned tempeh strips often use onion or garlic

**Use it:** Cubed in stir-fries; season strips with soy sauce and sesame oil and grill and use as an alternative to deli meat in sandwiches

FACTS

## Sharing the Microbiome Love: Poop Transplants

Another method that some doctors are using to help people reset the bugs in their gut is an ick-inducing procedure called fecal microbiota transplant (FMT), also referred to as fecal or stool transplantation—or, because why not, poop transplants. In FMT, the doctor takes a sample of stool from a person with a healthy gut and, during a colonoscopy or similar procedure, transfers the donor stool into the colon of a person with recurrent *C. difficile* colitis (*C. diff.*), a hard-to-get-rid-of complication that can occur from using antibiotics. The healthy person's poop takes over and diminishes the *C. diff.* while levels of good bugs increase; research finds fecal transplantation may be even more effective than antibiotics (remember, antibiotics take an almost opposite approach, killing off both bad and good). While the procedure is currently approved in the United States as an investigational therapy for patients with *C. diff.*, researchers are exploring its use in IBS and IBD—so you may be hearing more about it in the future. In the meantime, please, do not try it at home (you're laughing, but go ahead and google it—people DIY it. That is a really, really bad idea).

## Kimchi

As of this book's publication, kimchi, a Korean staple, had not yet been tested for FODMAP content. However, once you're in phase two of the plan, you can experiment with it as you would any other food. Start with a small amount (1 tablespoon) and work your way up to a full serving—it's typically used as a condiment, so 2 tablespoons should be plenty.

Use it: To add unique flavor to fried rice dishes; on the side of grilled meats

## Miso Paste

If you've ever eaten sushi, you've probably heard of miso soup—it's the translucent, salty broth usually served before your meal. When people refer to just "miso," however, they're talking about a Japanese seasoning paste typically made from fermented soybeans (the paste is mixed with broth to make the famous soup). Up to around 2 teaspoons is considered safe on a low-FODMAP plan.

**Look for:** Yellow and white misos, which are fairly mild in flavor, and red miso, which is more pungent. You can find them all in the refrigerated section of the supermarket or natural foods store, near the tofu.

**Use it:** In my Bowl o' Ramen recipe (page 171); whisked with lemon juice for an easy salad or rice bowl dressing

## Sourdough Bread

Some bakers make bread with yeast to help it rise more quickly. Others employ the traditional method of using sourdough culture (a mixture of bacteria and yeast) and good old-fashioned time to make the bread rise. Simple sourdough breads—even those made with wheat flour—have been measured to be low in FODMAPs (in moderation, of course). The sourdough culture actually eats the fructans, producing gas and helping the bread rise (much like what can happen in your gut!)—and cutting down on the level of FODMAPs in the bread as a result.

**Look for:** A sourdough bread made without honey or high-fructose corn syrup that does not contain any yeast in the ingredients—that gives you the clue that it's had a slow rise. Sourdough breads made from spelt or wheat are both considered OK.

**Use it:** In moderation. It's super exciting to realize there's a real bread you can safely have on a low-FODMAP plan. Just don't go all Texas Toast with sourdough (in other words, stay away from huge slices). Up to two thin slices (2 ounces/ 50 g total) is considered a serving.

# A WORD ABOUT PREBIOTICS

Another word you might hear getting tossed around is *prebiotics.* They are types of fibers that feed beneficial probiotic microorganisms in the gut. The research on taking prebiotic pills for IBS, however, is lacking. Some research shows that low doses might help, yet for some they can actually exacerbate symptoms—particularly for those with diarrhea-predominant IBS. Some prebiotic fibers are actually the very FODMAP carbohydrates that you avoid when you're Going Low. During phase one, it's probably best to minimize even food sources of prebiotic fiber; you'll slowly reintroduce them in phase two to assess what you can safely tolerate.

# CHAPTER 8

## The Gut-Brain Connection

**W**hile having IBS or another gut disorder puts your digestive tract at center stage, as we discussed in Chapter 2, your brain plays the supporting—but crucially important—role. It's sort of like when you get the dreaded "spinning wheel of death" on your computer (you know, the multicolored swirl that tells you "something does not compute"). You can clearly see that there's a problem on your screen; however, it's something deep inside the computer's programming that's making it freak out on you rather than the screen itself.

Communication from your brain to your gut works similarly to a never-ending group chat with your bestie: Your brain sends your gut messages, and your gut sends messages back, often at the same time. This channel—the Kik of your body, if you will—is called the gut-brain axis. Nerves that line the wall of the GI tract record information about how your gut is working and send the messages through the spinal cord and up to the brain. At the same time, the brain tells the gut how you're feeling emotionally—how stressed or relaxed you are, what you've been thinking about, and what's going on in other parts of your body. You tell your friend what's going on with you. She tells you how she's feeling. Sometimes you listen closely and respond to each other's every word. Other times you just keep yapping about your own day. But you're always, always talking—just like your brain and your gut.

# STRESS-RELATED SYMPTOMS

"I definitely get more stomachaches and sometimes even diarrhea from stress."

"Stress is probably the main factor in my IBS."

"[Stress] makes my symptoms a lot worse."

A person with IBS, it seems, may have a more active Kik chat than a person with a healthy gut. Whether motility—how quickly things move through the GI tract—is too fast (leading to diarrhea) or too slow (resulting in constipation), a person with IBS typically has more sensitivity to those sensations. As a result, the messages that get sent to the brain have way more angry-face emojis than those of a person without IBS.

There was a time when a person with IBS might hear from their doctor, "It's all in your head." Of course, now we know that there's much more to this debilitating disorder than not being very good at managing stress (you probably know this by now, but if your doctor says it's all in your head, it's a great time to find a new doctor). However, there's no doubt that emotions—while

not the cause of GI disorders—can play an important role in managing their symptoms. Of the teens and young adults that I interviewed for this book, 75 percent said that stress had a negative impact on their gut issues.

This book, of course, is all about doing everything you can to manage your condition. Just saying, "This sucks" doesn't help (even though it *does* suck— it truly, truly does—and sometimes you do need to get that off your chest). This is why I thought it was so important to give you ways to help smooth out the connections across that gut-brain axis. Brain-focused strategies are yet another tool you can have in your backpack— along with food and whatever probiotics, supplements, or medications your doctor suggests—to help you live your best life. Following are some stress busters for you to explore.

# EXERCISE

"I regret that workout," said no one ever. OK—so I got that off some motivational fitness person's Instagram. But it's true, I believe. Getting started with exercise is the hardest part. But once you've done it, you'll be so glad you challenged yourself, every time.

While the word *exercise* itself might conjure images of moms in workout gear or sweaty dudes from the football team getting ready for the big game, all it means is simply "activity requiring physical effort." In other words, the definition is pretty wide open—meaning everyone can find a form of exercise that appeals to them.

You're probably already aware that exercise is good for health in general. It strengthens your bones and muscles, boosts your immune power, helps keep you at a healthy weight, and is nature's best mood booster—the act of raising your heart rate causes the release of chemicals called endorphins, which work by activating receptors in the brain that reduce the perception of pain and just make you feel good. Breaking a sweat also helps diminish the release of stress hormones.

Between making you less sensitive to pain and curbing your nerves, it makes perfect sense that exercise could be a strategy in managing gut symptoms. When researchers in Sweden asked thirty-nine adults with IBS to increase their exercise level for twelve weeks, more than half had a reduction in symptoms; participants also went on to experience less depression and anxiety, and a better overall quality of life.

So what counts as exercise? Anything you can do that bumps your heart rate up for an extended period of time. How much should you get? Experts say teens (up to age seventeen) should aim for at least sixty minutes a day, five days a week; adults thirty minutes a day, five days a week. For some people (especially those who play sports), that comes naturally. For others, it seems totally unattainable—especially if gut problems have been getting in the way of your getting active.

If you're one of those people for whom exercise isn't already a regular part of your life, here's what I believe you should aim for: more. Don't get intimidated by recommendations to work up a sweat for at least an hour every school day. Maybe fifteen minutes a day is totally challenging for you. So that's where you start. When you get comfortable with that, strive for more.

## Anyone Can Exercise

You can do it. I promise. If you don't already have a form of exercise that speaks to you, here are a few to choose from: Running around a track, jogging around the neighborhood, walking in a shopping mall (no stopping for sales!), biking, spin class/ indoor cycling, Zumba class, swimming, dancing in your room with the door closed (or open—whatever!), working out with an app like Sworkit or Skimble, playing a sport that makes you break a sweat (bowling doesn't count), yoga (so good it gets its own section in this chapter), roller-skating (traditional or in-line), and so many more.

# MEDITATION

Ommmmmmm. . . . Excuse me, I heard the word *meditation* and immediately felt more relaxed. You see, meditation might sound a little "woo-woo," but it has proven benefits that give it plenty of credibility. Research shows it can help us better manage pain and stress—so it should come as no surprise that it can also help with gut problems.

When people with IBS took a class that focused on how emotions connect with symptoms (as you've learned in this book!) and taught relaxation and meditation techniques (and instructed participants to use them for fifteen minutes twice a day), they felt they had fewer symptoms and a better quality of life and were happier than people who didn't participate. Another study asked one half of a group of people with

inflammatory bowel disease to take a meditation workshop and put what they learned into practice, while the rest of the group took an educational seminar. Seven months later, the meditators had decreased their levels of C-reactive protein, a marker of inflammation in the body, while the people in the educational seminar stayed the same. Participants also reported fewer symptoms and said they felt better emotionally.

Convinced? Not quite? Here's my final selling point: Meditation is free, doesn't have to take up a lot of your time, and you can do it anywhere— and no one needs to know. Get started by going to a website like the UCLA Mindfulness Awareness Research Center (marc.ucla.edu/body.cfm?id=22) or downloading an app for your

## EXTRACURRICULAR ACTIVITIES

"I love my extracurriculars, so I have found myself able to muster up all of my energy to participate."

"I bring my own food to special events with my team."

"My parents enrolled me in every sport you can think of as a kid even though I had stomach issues, and it made me physically stronger and more confident."

smartphone like Calm or Headspace; all will walk you through exercises that will help you slow down and breathe, and maybe even diminish your symptoms.

## YOGA

While most types of yoga may not get your heart pumping in quite the same way an uphill run would, it's a better workout than you might think (although there are some exceptions; vinyasa and power yoga are two examples). If you've never taken a yoga class, you may have preconceived notions about twisting your body into complicated contortions. But yoga isn't just about being a human pretzel. It's a sequence of bends and exercises that help you link your breath to each and every movement. One of my former yoga teachers always called it *meditation in motion*, which sums it up

well. As you move your body, you learn to breathe, calm down, and let go.

Because exercise and meditation both have gut-health benefits, yoga, which essentially combines the two, is a winning option for you. When researchers at UCLA asked fourteen- to twenty-six-year-olds with IBS to take a yoga class twice a week for six weeks, nearly half reported a decrease in stomach pain, while around one third had a significant improvement in overall symptoms.

Bottom line on yoga: It's not a magic bullet, but there's a chance it may help—and it's great for other reasons, too. Research has linked it with helping teens manage emotions, improve self-esteem and attention span, and even get better grades! No harm in trying.

## SCHOOL EXAMS

"My exams officer knows about my IBS, so I'm allowed to go on toilet breaks.

"I always take time to go beforehand."

"Deep breathing helps me get through them."

"Last year I had to ask to go to the bathroom during finals. It was embarrassing, but they let me go."

# TALK THERAPY

Many of the teens I've spoken with about their experiences managing gut problems said that talking with someone who cares—a friend, relative, school counselor, or psychologist—was a big help to them. A review of forty-one studies from Vanderbilt University that looked at how well therapy helps digestive symptoms in adults with IBS supported the idea that talking can help decrease suffering and showed that the effects can last over the long term.

While it's fantastic if your mom, sister, or best friend can be that sounding board, I highly recommend talking to someone whose job it is to listen, like a psychologist or social worker. Professionals are trained in how to help people; they also take care to leave their feelings out of it (unlike a parent, who might have great intentions but feels wracked with guilt for passing the "bad belly" gene down to you). Another bonus is that the time with a therapist is *your* time—she won't be distracted by work deadlines or friends texting like a relative or friend might.

Remember, too, that there are real links between gut issues and conditions like depression, anxiety, and eating disorders. Having a GI issue doesn't mean you'll become depressed, of course, but you've undoubtedly got a lot on your plate—so there's every reason for you to take your emotional well-being seriously and make sure you are getting all the support you can.

## MANAGING STRESS

"I breathe in and out and remind myself that the stress will make my symptoms worse. I close my eyes and forget about everything."

"Meditation. It calms me."

"Talking about it with someone I trust."

"Coloring book, hanging out with friends, listening to music."

"My counselor taught me to focus on something around the classroom and describe whatever you're focusing on in your head. It sometimes takes your mind off your stomach."

# GUT-DIRECTED HYPNOTHERAPY

I must admit, I thought gut-directed hypnotherapy sounded a little wacky until I did some digging and found that there really is something to hypnotherapy—a.k.a. hypnosis— when it comes to managing gut symptoms. Hypnosis is a mental state in which a person is highly responsive to direction, and it naturally slows digestive function; a trained practitioner can use it therapeutically to help a patient decrease stress and improve GI function. A review article from Australia's Monash University reported that six out of seven studies on hypnotherapy found significant reductions in the uncomfortable effects of IBS, which were often maintained long after the hypnotherapy sessions ended. They also noted that it seemed to help patients with ulcerative colitis stay in remission from their symptoms.

So how do you find a certified hypnotherapist who will help you calm your gut and not make you cluck like a chicken? A good place to start is the American Society of Clinical Hypnosis (ASCH), a professional organization that requires members to have a graduate degree in a related health care discipline, a license or certification in the state in which they practice, and forty hours of approved hypnosis training, among other criteria. Their website, asch.net, can help you locate a practitioner in your area; your gastroenterologist or registered dietitian nutritionist may also be able to connect you with a practitioner she knows and trusts.

## GUT-DIRECTED BIOFEEDBACK

Biofeedback is a technique that trains people to control normally involuntary bodily functions like heart rate, blood pressure, and muscle tension. A therapist connects you to (painless) electrical sensors that receive messages about what's going on inside your body. As a signal like beeping or a flashing light briefs you on your inner workings, you work to change the way you think, feel, and act in order to change those rhythms. Research shows that biofeedback may be effective in people with constipation-predominant IBS, helping them to relax their pelvic floor muscles.

Because anyone can perform biofeedback in most states, it's important to make sure your biofeedback practitioner has adequate training and experience. Again, ask your GI doc or registered dietitian nutritionist if he has a trusted professional to refer you to. If not, the Biofeedback Certification International Alliance (bcia.org) is a professional organization that keeps a database of certified practitioners; make sure anyone you use is experienced in gut disorders as well as certified to provide biofeedback services.

# CHAPTER 9

# Go Low, Go Delicious:

## RECIPES

Embarking on a low-FODMAP diet can feel overwhelming, given the number of restrictions put in place. But Going Low doesn't have to mean going hungry. The great news is that there are still loads of delicious ingredients and food products you can enjoy while you're on a low-FODMAP plan. I've designed the breakfasts, lunches, dinners, and desserts in this chapter to be easy to prepare and so delicious that you'll forget all about the ingredients you can't have. Most of the recipes are vegetarian or easily vegetarian-adaptable, many are vegan, and all are gluten-free (as long as you use certified gluten-free ingredients), so they should suit the majority of your friends and family. (No worries if you're a proud carnivore; there are plenty of opportunities to eat some meat!)

# BELLY-BALANCING BREAKFASTS

# BANANA-BLUEBERRY SMOOTHIE

**SERVES 1 // PREP TIME: 3 MINUTES // COOK TIME: NONE**

No time for a sit-down breakfast? Throw these four ingredients into a blender and give it a whirl for a simple superfast morning meal you can toss in a to-go cup and sip on the way to school.

½ medium frozen banana

¼ cup (30 g) frozen blueberries

¾ cup (180 ml) unsweetened vanilla almond milk

½ cup (125 g) plain lactose-free yogurt

Place the banana, blueberries, milk, and yogurt in a blender and blend until smooth.

Per serving: 163 calories, 6.5 g fat (2.7 g saturated fat), 26 g carbs, 199 mg sodium, 2.5 g fiber, 6.5 g protein

# EGG FLOWERS

SERVES 1 // PREP TIME: 2 MINUTES // COOK TIME: 7 MINUTES

A childhood favorite of mine was egg-in-a-frame (also called picture-in-a-frame, egg-in-a-nest, and many other colorful names)—a comfort-food dish made by cutting a circle out of a slice of bread and cooking an egg in it. That still tastes pretty good to me and is perfect for a low-FODMAP plan if you make it with approved bread. These days, though, I prefer this colorful spin on the classic. By using ½-inch (13 mm) rings of bell pepper instead of bread, you add some produce to your meal, not to mention a little color and whimsy (Who wants flowers for breakfast?!). Try it on a morning when you have a little time to cook, or later in the day as a playful breakfast-for-dinner. These Egg Flowers are great on their own, with a slice of approved gluten-free bread, or with the Best-Ever Breakfast Potatoes on page 152 for a heartier meal.

**Nonstick cooking spray**

**Two ½-inch (13 mm) thick bell pepper rings, any color**

**2 eggs**

**Salt and pepper**

1. Spray a medium skillet with cooking spray and place over medium-low heat.

2. When the skillet is hot, put the pepper rings in the pan and crack one egg into each ring.

3. Cook until the whites begin to set, about 3 minutes.

4. Cover the pan and continue cooking until the yolks become firmer, an additional 2 to 3 minutes, or until the eggs are cooked to your preference.

5. Season with salt and pepper to taste.

Per serving: 158 calories, 9.5 g fat (3 g saturated fat), 3.7 g carbs, 144 mg sodium, 1 g fiber, 13 g protein

# HAPPY BELLY BREAKFAST TACOS

**SERVES 4 (2 TACOS EACH) // PREP TIME: 10 MINUTES // COOK TIME: 15 MINUTES**

A day that begins with tacos is a good day, in my opinion. Sadly, though, with the onion-packed pico de gallo, avocado-heavy guacamole, not to mention the beans, tacos are a pretty low-FODMAP-unfriendly choice. Here's what's great about breakfast tacos, though—the main attractions are the (low-FODMAP-approved) eggs. This taco recipe might be made for morning, but you can use it as a satisfying meal any time of day.

1 tablespoon plus 1 teaspoon vegetable oil

1 medium zucchini, diced

1 medium yellow squash, diced

Eight 6-inch (15 cm) soft corn tortillas

8 eggs

1/8 teaspoon salt

1/4 cup (5 g) chopped cilantro

1/4 cup (5 g) chopped scallions, green parts only

1/2 avocado, chopped

Go Low–approved hot sauce like Original Cholula

NOTE: One bunch of scallions from the grocery store is the gift that keeps on giving. Simply snip off the green parts (the only part you're allowed to use when you're Going Low) and plop the white roots into a cup of water. Keep the cup near a sunny window, changing the water daily so it stays fresh, and the green parts of the scallion will grow back. Snip them off and start over again, indefinitely!

1. Heat 1 tablespoon of the vegetable oil in a medium skillet or cast-iron pan over medium-high heat.

2. Add the zucchini and yellow squash and sauté until slightly browned, about 5 minutes. Meanwhile, heat a 10-inch (25 cm) skillet over medium heat and cook the tortillas in the dry pan, one by one, for 30 seconds on each side.

3. Place 2 tortillas on each of 4 plates and evenly distribute the squash mixture among the tortillas.

4. In a bowl, whisk the eggs and salt until well blended.

5. Using the skillet you used to warm the tortillas, heat the remaining 1 teaspoon of oil over medium heat. Add the eggs, stirring gently to scramble them, until no liquid remains in the skillet and the eggs appear firm and not runny, about 2 minutes. Divide the eggs evenly among the tortillas.

6. Garnish each serving with cilantro, scallions, avocado, and hot sauce to taste.

7. If you have any leftover ingredients, you can assemble them into tacos, roll up, wrap in aluminum foil, and microwave the next morning. (Don't forget to completely remove the foil before microwaving!)

Per serving: 345 calories, 19 g fat (7.5 g saturated fat), 28 g carbs, 272 mg sodium, 6 g fiber, 17 g protein

# BANANA BREAD OATMEAL

**SERVES 2 // PREP TIME: 1 MINUTE // COOK TIME: 12 MINUTES**

Few things make a kitchen smell better than freshly baked banana bread. Of course, if you're getting ready to head out the door for the day, there's hardly time for baking. That's why I created this easy peasy oatmeal recipe. It takes only around 15 minutes to throw together, but the scent is just as amazing. What's more, the bananas help bulk up the smallish low-FODMAP-approved oatmeal serving to give you a satisfying meal.

1 cup (240 ml) water

Pinch of salt

½ cup (50 g) rolled oats
  (certified gluten-free if
  necessary)

¼ cup (30 g) chopped walnuts

1 large ripe banana, thinly sliced

1 teaspoon coconut oil

¼ teaspoon vanilla extract

¼ teaspoon ground cinnamon

Up to ½ cup (120 ml)
  unsweetened almond milk

1. In a medium saucepan, bring the water and salt to a boil over high heat.

2. Add the oats and reduce the heat to medium-low. Simmer, uncovered, for about 4 to 5 minutes, until the water is absorbed.

3. While the oatmeal is cooking, heat a small skillet over low heat, add the walnuts to the dry pan, and cook, stirring constantly, to bring out their flavor, around 45 seconds. Remove from the heat and set aside.

4. Add the banana, coconut oil, vanilla, and cinnamon to the oatmeal. Mix vigorously with a fork so the banana pieces break down and the mixture reaches a thick oatmeal consistency.

5. Slowly stir in in the almond milk until the consistency of the oatmeal is to your liking.

6. Divide the oatmeal evenly into two bowls and top with the walnuts.

7. Store leftovers in a lidded microwave-safe bowl. When you're ready to eat, reheat it in the microwave and add extra almond milk as needed.

Per serving: 324 calories, 19 g fat (7 g saturated fat), 34 g carbs, 193 mg sodium, 5 g fiber, 7 g protein

# EGG MUFFINS

**SERVES 6 (2 MUFFINS EACH) // PREP TIME: 5 MINUTES // COOK TIME: 20 MINUTES**

Eggs are a great go-to on a low-FODMAP plan. And while it's not hard to make scrambled, poached, or fried eggs, all of those methods can take a little bit of practice to get right. That's why I wanted to create a fail-proof egg recipe that takes little time to master and less time at the stovetop. These egg muffins are my answer. All you need to do is chop up some low-FODMAP veggies, whisk some eggs, pour them into a muffin tin, and go. Eat them on their own or pair with my Best-Ever Breakfast Potatoes (page 152) or a slice of low-FODMAP toast like Udi's white bread for a satisfying meal.

**Nonstick cooking spray**

**12 eggs**

**¼ teaspoon salt**

**⅛ teaspoon pepper**

**1 cup chopped spinach (40 g) or kale (20 g)**

**½ cup (50 g) chopped red or orange bell pepper**

1. Preheat the oven to 350°F (180°C). Spray a 12-cup standard muffin pan with nonstick cooking spray.

2. In a medium bowl, whisk the eggs, salt, and pepper.

3. Distribute the spinach and bell pepper evenly in the prepared muffin cups.

4. Pour the egg mixture over vegetables, filling each cup at least halfway.

5. Bake for 20 minutes, or until the eggs have set completely and a toothpick inserted into the middle of the biggest muffin comes out clean.

6. Cool slightly before loosening each muffin with a table knife and popping them out of the pan.

7. Eat right away or store in the refrigerator in an airtight container for up to 3 days. Reheat in the microwave, or enjoy cold.

Per serving: 148 calories, 9.5 g fat (3.1 g saturated fat), 1.5 g carbs, 243 mg sodium, 0.2 g fiber, 12.5 g protein

# THE BEST-EVER BREAKFAST POTATOES

SERVES 4 // PREP TIME: 6 MINUTES // COOK TIME: 45 MINUTES

During the week, morning meals are all about speed and convenience. But when it's the weekend, I can't wait to take my time to make a proper breakfast, which almost always includes these two-step, superspecial breakfast potatoes. The "forking" technique ups the surface area, which makes the potatoes extra crunchy (the best part of breakfast potatoes, of course). And unlike the hash browns or home fries that may come with your eggs at the local diner, these are made to be Go Low friendly, so no onions, garlic, or anything else that might mess with your belly. Serve these beside any egg dish or make a simple but delish breakfast bowl by layering a serving of potatoes, a big handful of sautéed baby spinach, and one or two over-easy eggs.

**4 medium white potatoes**

**¼ cup (60 ml) olive oil**

**½ teaspoon salt, plus more to taste**

**¼ teaspoon pepper, plus more to taste**

**1 teaspoon dried or 1 tablespoon fresh chopped herbs (like rosemary or oregano)**

1. Bring a medium saucepan half filled with water to boil over a medium flame. Meanwhile, scrub the potatoes and cut them into 1-inch (2.5 cm) cubes. Add the potato cubes to the boiling water and cook until just soft enough to eat, around 10 minutes.

2. While you're waiting for the potatoes to cook, preheat the oven to 425°F (220°C).

3. Drain the cooked potatoes by placing a colander in the sink and carefully pouring the water and potatoes into it. When the potatoes are cool enough to handle, mix them around with a fork so the edges become jagged and softened.

4. Pour the potatoes onto a 9- x 13-inch (23 x 33 cm) baking sheet, drizzle them with the oil, and sprinkle on the salt and pepper. Bake for 30 to 45 minutes, turning every 10 minutes or so to ensure even cooking, until browned and crisp. Sprinkle the potatoes with herbs and with additional salt and pepper to taste.

5. Store leftovers in an airtight container for up to 3 days. Microwave or reheat in the oven at 200°F (95°C) (using the oven will help them stay crispy).

Per serving: 267 calories, 14 g fat (8 g saturated fat), 34 g carbs, 325 mg sodium, 5 g fiber, 3.5 g protein

# BELLY-BALANCING OVERNIGHT OATS

**SERVES 1 // PREP TIME: 5 MINUTES // CHILL TIME: OVERNIGHT**

When I'm scrolling through Pinterest, it seems like everybody is making a version of this breakfast. And why not? A few minutes of work at night and you have a satisfying and tasty meal ready to go for the morning rush. All you need to do to make this Go Low approved is use lactose-free yogurt and milk. Prep it in a mason jar with a lid so all you have to do is toss it in your bag on your way out the door.

⅓ cup (35 g) rolled oats (certified gluten-free if necessary)

⅓ cup (85 g) lactose-free plain yogurt

⅓ cup (80 ml) unsweetened almond milk

2 teaspoons chia seeds

1 tablespoon maple syrup

Pinch of salt

1 Put the oats, yogurt, milk, chia seeds, maple syrup, and salt in a bowl or jar with a lid. Mix well.

2 Cover and refrigerate overnight. Eat cold.

Per serving: 260 calories, 8 g fat (2 g saturated fat), 40 g carbs, 98 mg sodium, 5.9 g fiber, 8.3 g protein

**VARIATIONS:** One of the best things about overnight oats is that it's a simple canvas to which you can add your favorite flavors and textures. Here are some tried-and-true combinations you might like to add to your finished product before you chow down:

- ½ banana + 2 tablespoons peanut butter
- ¼ cup (30 g) blueberries + ¼ teaspoon cinnamon
- ¼ cup (45 g) raspberries + 1 tablespoon dark chocolate chips
- ½ cup (70 g) fresh pineapple cubes + 1 tablespoon unsweetened shredded coconut

# NO-BAKE PEANUT BUTTER BARS

**SERVES 16 // PREP TIME: 10 MINUTES // REFRIGERATION TIME: 1 HOUR OR MORE**

While nothing beats a satisfying breakfast at home, sometimes expecting people to squeeze in a sit-down morning meal is just not realistic. We've got school, work, trains to catch, people to see. Which is why I always keep a yummy bar or two in my purse for those moments when eating a meal is just not going to happen—and I recommend that my clients do the same. Sure, it's better to eat a so-called square meal, but it's better to eat a seminutritious bar than it is to stop for a doughnut before homeroom.

Unfortunately, if you're on a low-FODMAP plan, it can be hard to find a bar that meets your requirements. Many contain No foods like honey and dried fruit, leaving you with few options for phase one of the Go Low plan. These peanut butter bars help fill that need. Make up a batch and keep the extras in the fridge. Before hitting the road, toss one in your backpack so you'll have something for those "no time to eat, but I need something" moments. They also make a good between-classes snack.

Nonstick cooking spray

One 16-ounce (454 g) jar crunchy-style peanut butter

½ cup (120 ml) maple syrup

1½ cups (160 g) rolled oats (certified gluten-free if necessary)

½ cup (15 g) gluten-free brown rice cereal (like Erewhon's)

½ cup (90 g) pumpkin seeds

1. Spray a 9 x 11-inch (23 x 28 cm) glass baking dish with cooking spray.

2. In a medium bowl, whisk the peanut butter and maple syrup until combined.

3. With a rubber spatula, fold in the oats, rice cereal, and pumpkin seeds. As it gets harder to combine the ingredients, don't be afraid to get in there and use your hands!

4. Scrape the peanut mixture into the prepared pan and press firmly to compact the ingredients and make an even layer.

5. Place the dish in the refrigerator until the bars set, at least 1 hour.

6. Remove the dish from the refrigerator and cut into 16 equal pieces. Store the bars in individual plastic bags in the refrigerator or freezer for an easy grab-and-go snack or meal.

Per serving: 291 calories, 20 g fat (3 g saturated fat), 20.5 g carbs, 129 mg sodium, 1.3 g fiber, 11.5 g protein

# GO LOW BAKED PANCAKE

**SERVES 4 // PREP TIME: 5 MINUTES // COOK TIME: 20 MINUTES**

I adore pancakes; what I'm not a fan of is standing over the stove for a half hour waiting for all of them to cook. My solution is the baked pancake. I've made it even easier to do by combining the ingredients in a blender. Use a Go Low–approved gluten-free flour like Bob's Red Mill 1-to-1 or King Arthur Flour's gluten-free all-purpose baking mix, and you've got breakfast made— especially if you serve it with a side of berries and a dollop of lactose-free yogurt to balance out that plate.

2 teaspoons vegetable oil

3 eggs

¾ cup (180 ml) unsweetened almond milk

½ cup (60 g) gluten-free flour

2 teaspoons vanilla extract

1 tablespoon granulated sugar

Pinch of salt

1 tablespoon butter, chopped

Juice of ½ lemon

1 tablespoon powdered sugar

1. Preheat the oven to 425°F (220°C). Grease a 9-inch (23 cm) round cake pan or cast-iron skillet with the oil.

2. Place the eggs, milk, flour, vanilla, granulated sugar, and salt in a blender and blend until frothy, around 45 seconds.

3. Pour the pancake mix into the prepared pan and bake for 20 minutes, or until the pancake is puffy and lightly browned.

4. Remove from the oven and sprinkle with the butter. Cut the pancake into quarters (the puffiness will settle down as you do this) and serve each piece with a squeeze of lemon juice and a light dusting of powdered sugar.

5. Store leftovers in the refrigerator for up to 3 days; reheat in microwave or oven on low heat.

Per serving: 164 calories, 7.5 g fat (3 g saturated fat), 17 g carbs, 111 mg sodium, 1.5 g fiber, 6.5 g protein

# LIP-SMACKIN' LUNCHES

# CREAMY (BUT CREAM-FREE) TOMATO-BASIL SOUP

**SERVES 4 // PREP TIME: 5 MINUTES // COOK TIME: 50 MINUTES**

Being on a low-FODMAP plan can definitely limit your ability to eat your favorite comfort foods, which can feel like a total bummer. That's why I developed this easy FODMAP-friendly recipe for one of my ultimate comfort foods: cream of tomato soup. Throw this together on a rainy day, pair it with a grilled cheese sandwich made with gluten-free bread and cheddar cheese, and you won't feel one bit like you're missing out.

**6 medium tomatoes**

**¼ cup (60 ml) olive oil**

**¼ cup (35 g) macadamia nuts**

**5 medium basil leaves**

**1 teaspoon salt**

**1 cup (240 ml) water, plus more to soak nuts**

1. Preheat the oven to 375°F (190°C).

2. Coat the tomatoes with the olive oil and place on a baking sheet. Roast for 45 minutes, flipping once to ensure even cooking, until the tomato skins appear slightly browned and wrinkled.

3. While the tomatoes are roasting, place the macadamia nuts in a bowl and cover them with water.

4. When the tomatoes have finished roasting, drain the macadamia nuts in a colander and put them in a blender along with the roasted tomatoes, basil, salt, and 1 cup (240 ml) water. Blend on high until smooth, adding additional water as necessary to thin the soup to your desired consistency. The soup should be the right temperature to eat; if not, reheat on the stove or in the microwave.

5. Store any leftovers in an airtight container for up to 3 days and reheat in the microwave or on the stove.

Per serving: 213 calories, 20 g fat (3 g saturated fat), 8.3 g carbs, 591 mg sodium, 3 g fiber, 2.5 g protein

# CARROT AND CORIANDER SOUP

**SERVES 4 // PREP TIME: 5 MINUTES // COOK TIME: 50 MINUTES**

When I was a junior in college, I studied in London for a semester and lived in an apartment with three other girls. It was the first time I was living out of the dorms and cooking for myself, and I had a lot to learn. It took me years to realize that much of the culinary information I absorbed that semester had a British accent. Little did I know that the carrot and coriander soup I bought weekly in a box at Tesco actually contained the herb cilantro, which I've always associated with guacamole. In the United States, we use the word *coriander* to refer to the seeds of the plant and *cilantro* for the leaves, but in the UK it's all coriander. And now you know, too. Whatever you call it, this light soup will warm you up. It transports me to foggy London every time I make it.

---

1 pound (455 g) carrots

1 tablespoon olive oil

2 tablespoons plus 2 cups (480 ml) water

1 cup (240 ml) unsweetened almond milk

¾ teaspoon salt

¼ teaspoon ground nutmeg

1 tablespoon chopped fresh cilantro leaves

---

1 Preheat the oven to 400°F (200°C).

2 Scrub the carrots and trim off the tops. Place them in a roasting pan and drizzle them with the olive oil and 2 tablespoons of the water.

3 Roast for 45 minutes, tossing every 10 minutes to ensure even cooking, until the carrots have softened and slightly browned.

4 Place the carrots in a blender along with the 2 cups (480 ml) water, the milk, salt, nutmeg, and cilantro. Blend on high until smooth. The soup should be the right temperature to eat; if not, reheat it on the stove or in the microwave.

5 Store in an airtight container for up to 3 days. Reheat in the microwave or on the stove.

Per serving: 96 calories, 27 g fat (1 g saturated fat), 12 g carbs, 561 mg sodium, 3.5 g fiber, 1.5 g protein

# QUINOA TABBOULEH

This Middle Eastern salad is usually made with bulgur, a form of cracked wheat that the Monash University lab tested to be low FODMAP only in very small amounts. It's also typically made with low-FODMAP no-nos garlic and onions. I've tweaked the traditional recipe to make it Go Low friendly while still tasting delicious. Make a batch for the week; when you're ready to pack your lunch, toss it in a container on top of a handful of greens. Add in a protein of your choice, like grilled chicken, tuna, or ¼ cup (40 g) canned chickpeas, and you've got a meal.

1 cup (170 g) quinoa, rinsed well

2 cups (480 ml) water

1 teaspoon salt

2 large tomatoes, chopped

1 large cucumber, chopped

½ cup (10 g) chopped flat-leaf parsley

¼ cup (5 g) chopped mint

2 tablespoons chopped scallions, green parts only

Juice of 1 lemon

2 tablespoons olive oil

1 In a medium saucepan, combine the quinoa with the water and ½ teaspoon of the salt. Bring to a boil over medium-high heat, reduce the heat to low, and cover. Let simmer until the quinoa absorbs the water, about 15 minutes.

2 Turn off the heat and let the quinoa sit, covered, for another 5 minutes. Fluff it with a fork, then pour it into a large bowl.

3 Add the remaining ½ teaspoon of salt, the tomatoes, cucumber, parsley, mint, scallions, lemon juice, and olive oil. Toss well and serve or store in an airtight container for later.

Per serving: 167 calories, 6.5 g fat (1 g saturated fat), 23.3 g carbs, 99 mg sodium, 3.2 g fiber, 5 g protein

# VIETNAMESE NOODLE SALAD

### SERVES 4 // PREP TIME: 15 MINUTES // COOK TIME: 8 MINUTES

Don't be deceived by the long ingredients list: This recipe is simple to make and even easier to eat a big bowl full of. Thanks in part to a generous helping of fresh herbs like mint, basil, and cilantro, this taste bud–tingling recipe is the one to try if you're feeling like life without garlic and onions is destined for bland.

## DRESSING

¼ cup (52 g) packed brown sugar

¼ cup (60 ml) lime juice (freshly squeezed or store-bought)

3 tablespoons rice wine vinegar

2 tablespoons fish sauce

¼ teaspoon crushed red pepper flakes (more if you like it spicy)

¼ teaspoon minced fresh ginger

## SALAD

8 ounces (225 g) brown or white rice vermicelli noodles

1 medium head romaine lettuce

1 medium carrot, thinly sliced

1 medium cucumber, thinly sliced

1 teaspoon vegetable oil

12 ounces (340 g) peeled and deveined shrimp (about 24 medium), or one 14-ounce (397 g) package extra firm tofu, cut into 8 slabs

## GARNISHES

¼ cup (5 g) loosely packed fresh mint, chopped

¼ cup (5 g) loosely packed fresh cilantro, chopped

¼ cup (5 g) loosely packed fresh basil or Thai basil, chopped

2 tablespoons chopped scallions, green parts only

¼ cup (35 g) salted peanuts

1. **Make the dressing:** In a medium bowl, whisk the sugar, lime juice, vinegar, fish sauce, red pepper flakes, and ginger until well combined. Set aside.

2. **Make the salad:** Cook the vermicelli according to the package instructions. While the noodles are cooking, tear the lettuce into bite-size pieces and distribute among four bowls.

3. Drain the noodles and top each bed of lettuce with equal amounts of vermicelli noodles, carrot, and cucumber. Drizzle 3 tablespoons of the dressing over each salad.

4. Heat the oil in a large skillet over medium heat, then add the shrimp or tofu in a single layer so every piece is touching the pan. Cook until the shrimp are opaque throughout or the tofu is gently browned on each side, 3 to 4 minutes per side (use tongs to turn the shrimp or a spatula to flip the tofu).

5. **Garnish the salads:** While the shrimp or tofu is cooking, sprinkle 1 tablespoon each of the mint, cilantro, and basil on each salad. Distribute the hot shrimp or tofu evenly among the bowls on top of the noodles, then top each salad with ½ tablespoon of the scallions and 1 tablespoon of the peanuts.

Per serving (with tofu): 484 calories, 13 g fat (1.5 g saturated fat), 75 g carbs, 780 mg sodium, 10 g fiber, 20 g protein

# OPEN-FACE EGG MASH

**SERVES 1 // PREP TIME: 5 MINUTES // COOK TIME: NONE**

Sure, you could make some simple egg salad with mayo (no celery or onions), plop it between two slices of gluten-free bread, and call it a day. But that's kind of boring, don't ya think? I would much rather have this cool sandwich with a surprise topping to make it extra special. Serve with a side of veggies like sliced cucumbers or red bell pepper to balance out your plate.

2 hard-boiled eggs

1 to 2 tablespoons mayonnaise, to taste

Salt and pepper

2 slices gluten-free bread (like Udi's white sandwich bread), toasted

1 ounce (30 g) potato chips

Optional seasonings: low-FODMAP-approved hot sauce, smoked paprika

1 In a medium bowl, mash the eggs with a fork. Add the mayonnaise and salt and pepper to taste.

2 Divide the egg salad between the two slices of toast.

3 Crumble the chips over top and sprinkle on any optional seasonings.

Per serving: 545 calories, 31 g fat (5.5 g saturated fat), 49 g carbs, 752 mg sodium, 4 g fiber, 17.5 g protein

## HOW DO I MAKE A HARD-BOILED EGG?

This will come in handy on the low-FODMAP plan! To hard-boil eggs, place 6 eggs in a medium saucepan and cover them with cold water by about 1 inch (2.5 cm). Bring the water to a boil over medium-high heat. As soon as the water starts boiling, cover the pot, remove it from the heat, and set it aside for 10 minutes. Drain the eggs and then put them in an ice-water bath to cool. Remove the eggs from the water, peel, and you've got a snack or part of a meal ready to go.

# GO LOW GREEK SALAD

SERVES 1 // PREP TIME: 5 MINUTES // COOK TIME: NONE

I'm a New Yorker, born and bred, and I now live just across the border in New Jersey—which means eating at Greek-owned diners is basically in my DNA. But I had to travel all the way to Greece to realize that the Greek salads I grew up eating were pretty different from the typical salads there (for starters, most don't use lettuce). But whether you're talking about a traditional Greek *horiatiki* or an Americanized version, those Go Low–forbidden onions always play a prominent role. Not in my Go Low Greek Salad, though! Enjoy it for lunch on its own or share it with a friend as a starter for grilled fish and lemon potatoes, just like they do in Greece.

½ cup (65 g) chopped cucumber

1 small green bell pepper, chopped

1 small tomato, chopped

6 small olives

1 tablespoon chopped scallion, green parts only

1 tablespoon olive oil

1 teaspoon lemon juice (freshly squeezed or store-bought)

Salt and pepper

¼ cup (60 g) crumbled plain feta cheese

1 teaspoon dried oregano

1. Mix the cucumber, green pepper, tomato, olives, scallion, olive oil, and lemon juice in a medium bowl. Add salt and pepper to taste.

2. Sprinkle the feta and oregano on top and serve.

Per serving: 600 calories, 44 g fat (13 g saturated fat), 46 g carbs, 722 mg sodium, 6 g fiber, 10 g protein

# RAINBOW MASON JAR SALAD

**SERVES 1 // PREP TIME: 15 MINUTES // COOK TIME: NONE**

If the thought of bringing lunch to school gives you nightmares about smooshed peanut butter and jelly sandwiches, it's probably time you graduated from those little-kid brown-bag meals to something more mature. My pick? This salad in a mason jar—making it instantly portable, and so pretty you'll want to Instagram it. The recipe is suitable for vegetarians, but feel free to throw in some leftover chicken breast, shrimp, or sliced steak—or grilled tofu if you want to keep it vegetarian-friendly—to make it a heartier meal.

## DRESSING

**1 tablespoon olive oil**

**1½ teaspoons maple syrup**

**½ teaspoon lemon juice (freshly squeezed or store-bought)**

**⅛ teaspoon coarse-ground prepared mustard**

## SALAD

**1 radish, sliced thinly**

**1 small carrot, grated (shred it with a cheese grater, or buy grated carrots in a bag or at a salad bar)**

**⅓ medium yellow bell pepper, chopped**

**⅓ medium cucumber, chopped**

**¼ cup (30 g) blueberries**

**⅛ medium purple cabbage, thinly sliced (or ¼ cup/14 g preshredded cabbage)**

**¼ cup (30 g) crumbled goat cheese**

**1 teaspoon sunflower seeds**

**½ cup (65 g) packed baby kale**

1 **Make the dressing:** In a small bowl, whisk the oil, maple syrup, lemon juice, and mustard until well combined. Pour into a quart-size mason jar.

2 **Make the salad:** Stack the salad ingredients on top of the dressing in the order given: radish, carrot, yellow bell pepper, cucumber, blueberries, cabbage, goat cheese, sunflower seeds, and kale, which will both create a pretty rainbow effect and keep your salad from becoming soggy.

3 Keep the mason jar upright in a refrigerator or in a cooler bag until you're ready to eat it; when it's time to eat, turn the jar upside down and shake it to distribute the dressing throughout the salad. You can pour it into a bowl or eat it directly out of the jar.

Per serving: 485 calories, 33 g fat (14 g saturated fat), 33 g carbs, 313 mg sodium, 5 g fiber, 17 g protein

# SWEET 'N' SPICY CILANTRO-LIME CRUNCH BOWL

## SERVES 4 // PREP TIME: 10 MINUTES // COOK TIME: 20 MINUTES

Let's be honest: The right dressing and fun toppings make up about 95 percent of a salad's deliciousness. And if it's a Southwestern flavor you crave, the combination of. Sweet-n'-Spicy Lime Dressing with a sprinkle of crunchy and salty tortilla chips, chopped cilantro, creamy avocado (just a touch, to stay within Go Low limits!), and scallions can't be beat. Along with additional bite from fresh veggies and the toothsome texture and winning flavor of Cilantro-Lime Quinoa, this salad will fill you up and make you as happy as a dancing Bitmoji. For a heartier meal, add on a serving of grilled chicken, salmon, shrimp, tofu, or beef—the extra protein will give your meal a little more staying power.

### CILANTRO-LIME QUINOA

1 cup (170 g) quinoa, rinsed well

2 cups (480 ml) water

1 tablespoon chopped cilantro

2 teaspoons lime juice

### SWEET 'N' SPICY LIME DRESSING

¼ cup (60 ml) olive oil

2 tablespoons lime juice

2 tablespoons maple syrup

1 teaspoon salt

⅛ teaspoon ground chipotle powder

Pinch of cayenne pepper (more if you like a kick)

### SALAD

4 cups (140 g) chopped romaine lettuce

½ yellow bell pepper, chopped

½ orange bell pepper, chopped

12 cherry or grape tomatoes, chopped

### GARNISHES

1 cup (100 g) crushed tortilla chips

¼ cup (5 g) chopped cilantro

½ avocado, chopped

¼ cup (5 g) chopped scallions, green parts only

1 **Make the quinoa:** In a medium saucepan, combine the quinoa with the water. Bring to a boil over medium-high heat, reduce the heat to low, and cover. Let simmer until the quinoa is soft and the little "tails" are spiraling out from the seeds, about 15 minutes.

2 Remove the pan from the heat, mix in the cilantro and lime juice, and transfer the

quinoa to a large bowl and let cool to room temperature.

3 **Make the dressing:** While the quinoa is cooking, whisk the olive oil, lime juice, maple syrup, salt, ground chipotle, and cayenne pepper in a medium bowl until well blended. (You can also do this step in a food processor so it blends more thoroughly.) Set aside.

④ **Make the salad:** Put a quarter of the chopped romaine in each of four bowls. Top each with a quarter of the quinoa mixture. Then divide the yellow and orange bell peppers and cherry tomatoes evenly among the bowls. Sprinkle 2 tablespoons of dressing on each salad. Garnish each with equal amounts of the tortilla chips, cilantro, avocado, and scallions.

⑤ To store extras, assemble the vegetables and quinoa mixture in one airtight container and the keep the dressing and garnishes in other containers. Add the dressing and garnishes when you are ready to eat.

Per serving: 490 calories, 25 g fat (3.5 g saturated fat), 60 g carbs, 682 mg sodium, 8 g fiber, 9 g protein

# DELICIOUS DINNERS

# PESTO NOODLES AND ZOODLES

**SERVES 4 // PREP TIME: 10 MINUTES // COOK TIME: 45 MINUTES**

Not many foods scream *summer* more than pasta with basil-y pesto sauce, tomatoes, and zucchini. If you've ever grown vegetables in the backyard, you know that the main ingredients in that delicious dish all grow at the same time, often leaving gardeners with more than they can keep up with. It's a no-brainer, then, to have them join forces in one delicious dish. Usually, pesto is loaded with garlic; in this recipe I use garlic-infused oil to make it low FODMAP. I also roast the tomatoes to concentrate the flavor and add a punch of sweetness. As for the pasta, I've used both gluten-free spaghetti and zucchini "zoodles" to stretch the recipe and give you a bigger helping; you can use all zucchini if you're looking for a lighter option (or it's July and you have a ton of zucchini to use up).

**16 cherry or grape tomatoes, halved**

**1 tablespoon plus ¼ cup (60 ml) olive oil (regular or garlic-infused)**

**One 8-ounce (227 g) package gluten-free spaghetti**

**1 medium zucchini**

**2 cups (30 g) loosely packed basil leaves**

**¼ cup (55 g) pine nuts**

**¼ cup (60 ml) lemon juice**

**1 teaspoon salt**

1. Preheat the oven to 375°F (190°C).

2. Toss the tomatoes with 1 tablespoon of the olive oil and spread them on a baking sheet. Roast for 45 minutes, stirring every 5 to 10 minutes, until the tomatoes have browned and are slightly shriveled.

3. While the tomatoes are roasting, cook the pasta according to the package directions.

4. Cut the zucchini into thirds, then spiralize it using a vegetable spiralizer with the smallest spaghetti-size blade (if you don't have a spiralizer, carefully slice the zucchini into thin strips using a sharp knife or a vegetable peeler). Set the zucchini noodles aside.

5. Place the remaining ¼ cup (60 ml) olive oil, the basil, pine nuts, lemon juice, and salt in a food processor. Process until thoroughly combined.

6. When the pasta is almost finished cooking, carefully drop the zucchini noodles into the boiling water. Stir thoroughly so the zucchini becomes gently softened in the water, about 30 seconds to 1 minute.

7. Drain the pasta and zucchini in a colander. Return it to the empty pot and add the basil mixture and tomatoes. Mix well and divide among four bowls.

*Recipe continues . . .*

8 Store leftovers in an airtight container for up to 3 days, then microwave to reheat or enjoy cold.

Per serving: 440 calories, 25 g fat (3 g saturated fat), 53 g carbs, 592 mg sodium, 8 g fiber, 6.5 g protein

## SPIRALIZE IT!

I'm not a big fan of kitchen gadgets—in my book, why would you waste space storing an apple slicer, cherry pitter, and bagel cutter when you can just use a knife? But there is one cooking tool that I've made room for in my small kitchen over the past few years, and I couldn't be more pleased to have it: the spiralizer. This little gadget allows you to hand crank any vegetable into long noodles of varying thickness. Veggie noodles don't exactly take the place of pasta, but they do make it a heck of a lot more fun to get a serving of produce in. There are several brands (including some electric ones); check out consumer reviews on sites like Amazon to decide which is right for you.

# EASY SALMON BURGERS

SERVES 4 // PREP TIME: 5 MINUTES // COOK TIME: 10 MINUTES

These four-ingredient, easy-to-make salmon burgers are perfect for nights when you've got nothing in the fridge and wish you could order a pizza. It's easy to keep the components on hand, and they take no time at all to make. The base recipe is delicious as is, but you can experiment with mixing in various low-FODMAP ingredients, such as grated carrots, grated ginger, chopped parsley, and more, to add nutrients and vary the flavor profile.

Two 6-ounce (170 g) cans wild salmon

1 egg

¼ cup (40 g) gluten-free bread crumbs, like Ian's Gluten-Free Original Panko

¼ teaspoon dried dill

Nonstick cooking spray

Optional: gluten-free low-FODMAP bread, lettuce leaves, tomato slices, mustard, and mayonnaise for serving

1. Place the salmon in a medium bowl and flake it with a fork until its consistency is even.

2. Add the egg, bread crumbs, and dill and mix until thoroughly combined.

3. Use your hands to mold the mixture into four patties.

4. Spray a large skillet with cooking spray and heat over medium heat. Place the patties in the hot skillet, working in batches if they won't all fit.

5. Cook the patties until lightly browned, 3 to 5 minutes on each side.

6. Serve each on bread, between two romaine or Boston lettuce leaves, or naked on a plate. Depending on your preference, top with mustard, mayonnaise, or both, as well as lettuce (if you haven't used lettuce as your "bread," that is) and tomato. Wrap leftover cooked burgers in foil or store in an airtight container in the fridge for up to 2 days.

Per serving (without optional ingredients): 108 calories, 3 g fat (0.5 g saturated fat), 8 g carbs, 219 mg sodium, 0.5 g fiber, 12 g protein

# LET US EAT LETTUCE WRAPS

**SERVES 4 // PREP TIME: 10 MINUTES // COOK TIME: 10 MINUTES**

Scientific fact: People love eating with their hands (OK, it's not scientific—but don't you think it's true?). This Asian-inspired chicken or tofu dish (use whichever you and your family prefer) is refreshing, satisfying, and most important, super fun to eat. The bean sprouts you'll sprinkle on top may not be a typical grocery purchase for your family, but you'll recognize them from restaurant dishes like pad Thai and Asian-inspired chicken salads. Get your napkins ready.

1 head butter lettuce

2 teaspoons canola oil

1 teaspoon garlic-infused olive oil

⅛ teaspoon red pepper flakes

1 pound (455 g) ground chicken or one 14-ounce (397 g) block extra firm tofu, chopped

2 tablespoons soy sauce or tamari

1 tablespoon rice wine vinegar

1 tablespoon sesame oil

One 8-ounce (227 g) can water chestnuts, drained and chopped

¼ cup (5 g) chopped scallions, green parts only

1 tablespoon minced fresh ginger

½ cup (50 g) bean sprouts

¼ cup (35 g) chopped peanuts

1 Separate the lettuce leaves; rinse and set aside.

2 In a large skillet, heat both the canola and garlic-infused oils over medium heat. Add the red pepper flakes and chicken or tofu, stirring until the chicken is cooked through and juices run clear—about 6 minutes. Drain any liquid or grease that remains.

3 Add the soy sauce, rice wine vinegar, sesame oil, water chestnuts, scallions, and ginger to the pan. Cook, stirring occasionally, for another 3 minutes.

4 Distribute the mixture on the reserved lettuce leaves, using the biggest leaves first; sprinkle each with bean sprouts and peanuts, and serve. To eat, hold the leaves with the toppings wrapped up inside.

Per serving (with chicken): 334 calories, 21 g fat (4 g saturated fat), 25 g carbs, 603 mg sodium, 2 g fiber, 26 g protein

# BOWL O' RAMEN

SERVES 4 // PREP TIME: 5 MINUTES // COOK TIME: 20 MINUTES

Who doesn't love slurping up a big bowl of noodles on a cold winter day? But there are two issues when it comes to those blocks of ramen you buy five for a dollar at the store: First, they're not low FODMAP, and, second, they're pretty unhealthy—loaded with sodium and heart-unhealthy saturated fat. Luckily, homemade—and better-for-you—bowls of ramen are becoming popular in restaurants across the United States (they've long been a mainstay in Japan, where ramen originated). Even so, between the onions and mushrooms often used to make broth, not to mention the wheat-based noodles, there's not much room for ramen on a low-FODMAP diet. That's why I created this recipe. It also happens to be vegetarian and can easily be made vegan (just use extra soy sauce in place of the fish sauce). Oh, and if you want meat in your soup, you can swap shredded chicken for the tofu.

2 tablespoons miso paste

5¼ cups (1.25 L) water

2 tablespoons low-sodium soy sauce or tamari (certified gluten-free if necessary)

1 tablespoon sesame oil

1 teaspoon fish sauce or extra soy sauce

¼ teaspoon red pepper flakes

5 ounces (140 g) Go Low–approved ramen noodles, like Lotus Foods Millet and Brown Rice Ramen

1 cup (40 g) baby spinach

One 14-ounce (397 g) block extra firm tofu, cubed

1 medium carrot, chopped

1 medium zucchini, chopped

¼ cup (5 g) chopped scallions, green parts only

1. In a stockpot over medium heat, whisk the miso paste and ¼ cup (60 ml) water until combined.

2. Add the 5 cups (1.2 L) water, the tamari, sesame oil, fish sauce, and red pepper flakes and bring to a boil. Reduce the heat to low and simmer for 15 minutes.

3. While the broth is simmering, prepare the ramen according to the package directions. Drain the cooked noodles and divide them evenly among 4 bowls. Top each bowl of noodles with an equal amount of spinach.

4. Right before you're ready to serve the soup, carefully add the tofu, carrot, and zucchini to the broth and simmer for about 5 minutes.

5. Evenly distribute the soup among the 4 bowls and garnish each with 1 tablespoon of scallions.

Per serving: 431 calories, 12 g fat (1.5 g saturated fat), 55 g carbs, 833 mg sodium, 7 g fiber, 21 g protein

# MINI POLENTA PIZZAS

**SERVES 1 // PREP TIME: 5 MINUTES // COOK TIME: 28 MINUTES**

These mini pizzas are easy to make; they also taste great and are fun to eat—perfect for a night when you're on your own for dinner or the rest of your family is eating something that's off-limits. Ready-to-eat polenta is a versatile ingredient that works well crisped up to use as a pint-size pizza crust. Serve these little pizzas with a side salad to balance out your plate.

Half 18-ounce (255 g) log prepared polenta

Nonstick cooking spray

½ cup (120 ml) low-FODMAP marinara sauce or canned chopped tomatoes

½ cup shredded mozzarella cheese

Optional toppings: ¼ cup (30 g) cubed chicken breast, ¼ cup (30 g) sliced black or green olives, ¼ cup (35 g) chopped pineapple, ¼ cup (55 g) sliced canned mushrooms (see note), ¼ cup (20 g) chopped eggplant, sautéed.

NOTE: Fresh mushrooms are high FODMAP, but canned ones are OK.

1 Preheat the oven to 375°F (190°C). Spray a baking sheet with cooking spray.

2 Slice the polenta into ½-inch (1.25 cm) rounds and place on the prepared baking sheet.

3 Bake for 25 minutes, flipping once halfway through, or until lightly browned on both sides. Carefully remove the baking sheet from the oven.

4 Preheat the broiler.

5 Spoon a bit of sauce and a sprinkle of cheese on each slice of polenta. Add optional toppings if using.

6 Broil the pizzas 1 to 2 minutes, until the cheese has melted.

Per serving (without additional toppings): 240 calories, 15.5 g fat (6 g saturated fat), 12.5 g carbs, 687 mg sodium, 1.5 g fiber, 12 g protein

# FAST FODMAP-FRIENDLY FRIED RICE

**SERVES 4 // PREP TIME: 5 MINUTES // COOK TIME: 12 MINUTES**

Chinese takeout is greasy and yummy and an easy way to put dinner on the table quickly. What those little white boxes cannot always give you, however: a low-FODMAP, health-boosting meal. That's why I love to whip up this fried rice when I think I have no time to cook—it's safe for anyone on a low-FODMAP plan, and it's full of nutritious, energizing ingredients. Plus, it comes together in just a few minutes. To make it extra easy, some companies sell frozen brown rice—you can quickly microwave it before adding it to the recipe to speed up your meal prep that much more. Take that, takeout!

1 tablespoon garlic-infused olive oil

1 teaspoon sesame oil

1 medium zucchini, finely chopped

1 small carrot, finely chopped

½ yellow bell pepper, finely chopped

1 egg, beaten

4 cups (720 g) cooked brown rice

12 ounces (340 g) cooked chicken breast, chopped, or 7 ounces (200 g) extra firm tofu, cubed

2 tablespoons soy sauce or tamari (certified gluten-free if necessary)

1 teaspoon liquid smoke

¼ cup (5 g) chopped scallions, green parts only

1. Warm the olive and sesame oils in a large skillet over medium heat. Add the zucchini, carrot, and bell pepper and cook, stirring, until just softened, about 2 minutes.

2. Push the vegetables off to the sides of the pan and pour the egg into the empty center. Stir the egg around with a rubber spatula so it scrambles as it cooks.

3. When the egg no longer looks wet, after about 2 minutes, stir everything in the pan until combined. Add the rice, chicken or tofu, soy sauce, and liquid smoke. Increase the heat and stir-fry until well combined and heated through, about 5 minutes.

4. Divide the rice evenly among 4 bowls and top each with 1 tablespoon of the scallions.

Per serving: 425 calories, 10 g fat (2 g saturated fat), 50 g carbs, 717 mg sodium, 5 g fiber, 33 g protein

# THAI QUINOA BOWL

SERVES 4 // PREP TIME: 8 MINUTES // COOK TIME: 15 MINUTES

Peanut sauce is ubiquitous in Thai food (meaning, it's everywhere)—and that may be the main reason I like the cuisine. Sweet, salty, creamy, and nutty—this dressing takes peanut butter to the next level. For this bowl-based meal, I took the basic peanut-sauce-topped predinner salad served at my favorite neighborhood Thai restaurant and transformed it into a hearty low-FODMAP dish. (You can also bulk it up by adding sliced chicken, steak, or tofu.) I love the way this meal tastes, of course, but I'm also a big fan of the fact that you can prep the various pieces of it (quinoa, hard-boiled egg, chopped veggies, peanut sauce) ahead of time and just toss them together when you're ready to eat. Not sure how to make hard-boiled eggs? It's easy, and a great basic cooking skill to have in your repertoire. See how on page 161.

1 cup (170 g) quinoa, rinsed well

2 cups (480 ml) water

1 teaspoon salt

1 cup (240 ml) canned coconut milk

½ cup (200 g) peanut butter

2 tablespoons brown sugar

1 tablespoon rice wine vinegar

Juice of ½ lime

½ red bell pepper, thinly sliced

2 cups (170 g) finely shredded red cabbage

4 hard-boiled eggs, sliced

¼ cup (5 g) chopped fresh cilantro

¼ cup (5 g) chopped scallions, green parts only

1. Combine the quinoa, water, and ½ teaspoon of the salt in a medium saucepan. Bring to a boil over medium-high heat, reduce the heat to low, and cover. Simmer until the quinoa is fluffy, about 15 minutes.

2. While the quinoa cooks, prepare the dressing. Place the coconut milk, peanut butter, brown sugar, rice wine vinegar, lime juice, and the remaining ½ teaspoon salt in a blender. Blend on high until well mixed.

3. Divide the quinoa evenly among 4 bowls. Top each with equal amounts of red bell pepper, red cabbage, and egg slices. Drizzle each bowl with about ¼ cup (60 ml) dressing and garnish with cilantro and scallions.

Per serving: 545 calories, 33 g fat (15 g saturated fat), 50 g carbs, 643 mg sodium, 4.5 g fiber, 18 g protein

# DECONSTRUCTED SUSHI BOWL

SERVES 1 // PREP TIME: 5 MINUTES // COOK TIME: NONE (UNLESS YOU HAVE TO COOK THE RICE)

I love sushi! But sadly, I'm more likely to spend dinnertime at home in pajamas trying to make a deadline and watching Netflix than I am out with friends at a glamorous sushi restaurant. That's why I invented this super-easy sushi bowl so I can always have the flavor of sushi at home—it also happens to cost a fraction of the price. I'm writing this as a one-serving recipe so you can make it for yourself on nights when your family is eating something high in FODMAPs. If they're jealous (and they will be!), simply multiply by as many servings as you'd like so the whole crew can enjoy it.

1 cup (180 g) cooked short-grain brown or white rice

3 ounces (85 g) smoked salmon, sliced into bite-size pieces

½ medium cucumber, chopped

2 sheets nori, crumbled

1 teaspoon sesame seeds

1 tablespoon soy sauce or tamari (certified gluten-free if necessary), optional

1 teaspoon wasabi paste, optional

1 Spoon the rice into a bowl.

2 Top with the smoked salmon, cucumber, nori, and sesame seeds.

3 Garnish with soy sauce and/or wasabi paste, if desired.

Per serving (not including optional ingredients): 468 calories, 12.4 g fat (2.3 g saturated fat), 55 g carbs, 129 mg sodium, 2 g fiber, 10 g protein

## FREEZING TIP

I love to keep a bag of prepackaged frozen rice on hand to make meals like this come together in no time at all. I buy mine at Trader Joe's or Whole Foods; the brand Birds Eye also makes it, and it's available at many grocery stores.

# DELICIOUS DESSERTS AND SUPER SNACKS

# BUCKWHEAT CREPES

### SERVES 4 (2 CREPES EACH) // PREP TIME: 10 MINUTES
### PLUS 1 HOUR FOR BATTER TO REST // COOK TIME: 30 MINUTES

These crepes are nutritious, easy to make, and great to keep on hand because they can be used as a base for meals and snacks, sweet or savory. I'm partial to crepes for dessert, which is why I put them in this section of the book. However, what I especially love is that you can make a batch of these crepes and keep them in the fridge for a few days; simply microwave or pan-heat one or two when you're hungry, topping as you see fit (see the table on the next page for ideas).

3 eggs

2 cups (480 ml) unsweetened almond milk

1 cup (120 g) buckwheat flour

1 cup (120 g) oat flour (you can make your own; see DIY Oat Flour)

½ teaspoon salt

Nonstick cooking spray

1. Whisk the eggs in a large bowl. Add the milk and blend thoroughly. Add the buckwheat flour, oat flour, and salt, mixing to combine. Cover and let the batter sit in the refrigerator for 1 hour. (If you're short on time, it's OK to skip this step.)

2. Spray a medium skillet with nonstick cooking spray and heat over high heat. Add ¼ cup (60 ml) batter to the pan, then roll the pan in a circular motion to make a very thin pancake. Cook until the batter sets, about 1 minute, then flip the crepe with a spatula and cook until firm on both sides, about 30 seconds.

3. Repeat with the remaining batter, stacking each crepe on a plate. When you're ready to eat, top each crepe with your desired ingredients. Roll the crepe up with the ingredients inside, and eat it with a knife and fork.

Per serving (not including any fillings): 278 calories, 8 g fat (2 g saturated fat), 39 g carbs, 446 mg sodium, 5 g fiber, 13 g protein

*Recipe continues . . .*

| MEAL | FILL WITH |
| --- | --- |
| Savory breakfast | Sunny-side-up egg + ¼ cup (10 g) baby spinach + 1 tablespoon grated Parmesan |
| Sweet breakfast | ¼ cup (65 g) lactose-free plain yogurt + ¼ cup (30 g) blueberries |
| Lunch | 2 slices smoked salmon + 2 tablespoons crumbled goat cheese + ¼ cup (10 g) baby arugula |
| Dinner | 3 ounces (85 g) chopped grilled chicken breast + ¼ cup (25 g) each sautéed fennel and red bell pepper |
| Fancy dessert | 2 tablespoons melted dark chocolate chips + ½ medium banana, sliced |
| Simple dessert | Lemon juice + 1 tablespoon maple syrup |

# DIY OAT FLOUR

Oat flour is a great ingredient for wheat-free cooking; it's also very easy to make if you don't have any on hand. Simply put some rolled oats in a blender or food processer and give them a whirl. In about 30 seconds, you'll have oat flour. Fun fact: Pulverized oats measure out roughly the same amount as rolled oats, so you can measure once and be done.

# SUPER-SEEDY RASPBERRY-CHIA JAM

**SERVES 8 // PREP TIME: 2 MINUTES // COOK TIME: 5 MINUTES**

Peanut butter and jam . . . toast and jam . . . what *doesn't* jam go with? Well, a low-FODMAP plan, because many jams and jellies you'll find at grocery stores are made with gut-unfriendly fruit juice like pear and apple, or sweeteners like high-fructose corn syrup. In this recipe, I blend Go Low–friendly raspberries and chia seeds in an easy-to-make, nutritious jam perfect for topping sandwiches, oatmeal, crepes, and more.

One 12-ounce (340 g) package frozen raspberries

2 tablespoons plus 1 teaspoon chia seeds

1 tablespoon sugar

Juice of ¼ lemon (about 2 teaspoons)

1. Pour the frozen berries into a medium saucepan and warm them over medium heat. When the berries are thawed and soft, mash them with a fork or spoon until they resemble a sauce or puree (you'll still see the seeds) and begin to bubble.

2. Reduce the heat to low and add the chia seeds, sugar, and lemon juice; stir until combined.

3. Allow the jam to simmer until the flavors blend, about 1 minute. Enjoy immediately as a topping or let cool, pour into a jar, cover, and store in the refrigerator.

Per serving: 40 calories, 1.5 g fat (0 g saturated fat), 6.5 g carbs, 1 mg sodium, 3 g fiber, 1 g protein

# BLUEBERRY-LEMON FROZEN YOGURT POPS

**MAKES 6 POPS // PREP TIME: 5 MINUTES // FREEZE TIME: 6 HOURS**

Who doesn't like a cold treat on a hot day? But with creamy frozen desserts off-limits when you're on a low-FODMAP plan, just hearing the ice cream truck come down the street can make you sad. Instead, put a batch of my Blueberry-Lemon Frozen Yogurt Pops in the freezer so you can have a cool snack on hand for when the mood strikes or you hear the sweet strains of the ice cream truck in the distance. These pops are made with (lactose-free, of course) yogurt and kefir, so they're loaded with healthy probiotic bacteria, meaning you can even eat them for breakfast. Ice pop molds cost just a few dollars and are available at stores like Target, Walmart, and Bed Bath & Beyond.

1 cup (120 ml) lactose-free kefir

1 cup (250 g) plain lactose-free, full-fat yogurt

½ cup (55 g) frozen blueberries, plus extra for optional garnish

2 tablespoons maple syrup

1 tablespoon chia seeds

1 teaspoon lemon juice

1. Place the kefir, yogurt, ½ cup blueberries, maple syrup, chia seeds, and lemon juice in a blender and blend until smooth and the chia seeds are no longer visible, about 1 minute.

2. Pour into ice pop molds, tapping the sides to remove some of the bubbles. If you want to be fancy, sprinkle a few extra blueberries into each mold so you'll have whole blueberries floating around in your yogurt pops.

3. Put the molds in the freezer and leave them until the pops are solid, about 6 hours, or overnight.

Per pop: 68 calories, 1.3 g fat (0 g saturated fat), 12 g carbs, 27 mg sodium, 1.5 g fiber, 2.5 g protein

# PEANUT BUTTER–CHOCOLATE POWER BALLS

**SERVES 6 (2 BALLS EACH) // PREP TIME: 5 MINUTES // CHILL TIME: 30 MINUTES**

I absolutely love the combination of peanut butter and chocolate. But many snacks and desserts that star this winning pair—like Reese's Peanut Butter Cups and Girl Scout Tagalongs—are not Go Low approved; they're also not nearly satisfying enough to power you through your algebra homework. That's why I love making these Peanut Butter–Chocolate Power Balls. The real peanut butter and chia seeds provide heart-healthy fats and satiating protein, the oats and coconut add filling fiber, and the chocolate and maple syrup make it a treat—in other words, they satisfy a sweet craving and keep your energy level up, all in low-FODMAP amounts.

½ cup (200 g) peanut butter

2 tablespoons maple syrup

½ teaspoon vanilla extract

1 cup (105 g) rolled oats

3 tablespoons dried shredded coconut

2 tablespoons dark chocolate chips

1 tablespoon chia seeds

1 Whisk the peanut butter, maple syrup, and vanilla in a medium bowl until combined.

2 Mix in the oats, 2 tablespoons of the shredded coconut, the dark chocolate chips, and chia seeds.

3 Scoop out 1 heaping tablespoon of the mixture, roll it into a ball, and place it on a baking sheet or in an ovenproof baking dish. Repeat to make a total of 12 balls. Sprinkle the balls with the remaining 1 tablespoon of coconut, turning them so they have coconut on all sides.

4 Put them in the refrigerator and chill for at least 30 minutes. For longer storage, use an airtight container and eat within a week.

Per serving: 261 calories, 16 g fat (4.3 g saturated fat), 27 g carbs, 13 mg sodium, 3 g fiber, 8 g protein

# EASY PEASY CHIA PUDDING

**SERVES 4 // PREP TIME: 10 MINUTES // CHILL TIME: 1 HOUR OR MORE**

Chia pudding seems to be everywhere, and it's no surprise—it's delicious, easy to make, and nutritious. And if you make it with the right ingredients, it's also perfect for a low-FODMAP treat or even breakfast. One of my favorite things about chia pudding is what a great canvas it makes for your creativity in the kitchen. This recipe makes a simple chia pudding that you can enjoy on its own, or let your imagination run wild by mixing or topping it with other Go Low–approved ingredients like berries, dried shredded coconut (no more than ¼ cup/20 g), peanut butter, cinnamon, nutmeg, mint, cocoa powder, and bananas.

**2 cups (480 ml) unsweetened almond milk**

**2 tablespoons maple syrup**

**¼ teaspoon vanilla extract**

**Pinch of salt**

**½ cup (50 g) chia seeds**

1. In a medium bowl, whisk the milk, maple syrup, vanilla extract, and salt until combined. Stir in the chia seeds and let the mixture sit for 5 minutes.

2. Whisk the mixture again to prevent the seeds from clumping and allow it to sit another 5 minutes.

3. Whisk the mixture again to break up any clumps, cover the bowl, and refrigerate for at least 1 hour. Before refrigerating, you can divide the pudding into 4 individual containers, like small mason jars, for ready-to-go snacks.

4. . Eat plain or mix in some of the suggested toppings.

Per serving: 168 calories, 9 g fat (1 g saturated fat), 18 g carbs, 98 mg sodium, 9 g fiber, 5 g protein

# CHOCOLATE-COVERED STRAWBERRY SHAKE

### SERVES 1 // PREP TIME: 5 MINUTES // COOK TIME: NONE

Berries dipped in chocolate make a winning combination. This shake puts the flavors of a rich chocolate-covered strawberry in a drink. The addition of a frozen banana makes it extra creamy; whenever bananas at my house start to turn brown, I peel them, pop them in a plastic bag, and freeze them so I can make a smoothie like this one whenever the mood strikes. Toss in a handful of spinach for extra nutrition.

1 small frozen banana

¾ cup (180 ml) lactose-free milk or unsweetened almond milk

½ cup (125 g) plain lactose-free yogurt

¼ cup (70 g) frozen strawberries

2 teaspoons cocoa powder

Place the banana, milk, yogurt, strawberries, and cocoa powder in a blender. Blend until smooth.

Per serving: 215 calories, 7 g fat (3 g saturated fat), 35 g carbs, 200 mg sodium, 5 g fiber, 7.5 g protein

# FROZEN BANANA BITES

**SERVES 6 (4 BITES EACH) // PREP TIME: 2 MINUTES // COOK TIME: 10 MINUTES**
**FREEZE TIME: 1 HOUR**

My family and friends love these Frozen Banana Bites so much, I can't make them fast enough! Banana seems to taste even creamier after it's been frozen, so the combination of frozen banana and chocolate is extra delicious. Just remember that you can eat only four of these in one sitting (otherwise, you'll be eating too much chocolate for the low-FODMAP plan. It can be easy to overdo something so delicious (especially a food that you can justify because it's mainly fruit). This recipe calls for a double boiler. If you don't have one, see What's a Double Boiler? on the next page for how to improvise. And make sure you have some wax paper on hand before you get started!

**½ cup (90 g) dark chocolate chips**

**1 teaspoon coconut oil**

**3 bananas**

1. Line a baking sheet with waxed paper.

2. Fill the bottom of a double boiler with about 1 inch (2.5 cm) of water and heat over medium heat. Pour the chocolate chips and coconut oil into the top of the double boiler and let melt, stirring every so often, until smooth and blended. Remove from the heat.

3. While the chocolate is melting, cut each banana into 8 round discs for a total of 24 slices (to make it easy, cut each banana in half horizontally, and then each half into four slices).

4. Carefully dip each banana slice roughly two-thirds of the way into the melted chocolate. Shake off the excess chocolate, then place the banana slice on the wax paper.

5. Put the baking sheet in the freezer for at least 1 hour. Once the banana bites are thoroughly frozen, you can store them in a resealable plastic bag.

Per serving: 159 calories, 7.5 g fat (4.6 g saturated fat), 25 g carbs, 0.5 mg sodium, 3 g fiber, 2 g protein

# WHAT'S A DOUBLE BOILER?

When a saucepan sits directly on a burner, the temperature is too hot for chocolate—try to melt chocolate that way and it will burn (and smell pretty nasty). A double boiler, a pot that's heated by steam from another pot below it, is the solution to that problem. Here's how you can make your own if you don't have one: Pour about 1 inch (2.5 cm) of water into a medium saucepan. Nestle a Pyrex bowl on top of the pan; use a bowl that fits snugly in the pan without touching the water below. Put the saucepan on the stove and heat the water; the steam will gently heat the contents of the bowl above. Because the temperature increases slowly, you'll be able to melt chocolate without burning it.

# OLIVE OIL AND HERB STOVETOP POPCORN

## SERVES 2 // PREP TIME: 1 MINUTE // COOK TIME: 5 MINUTES

Microwave popcorn is fine, sure—but once you see how easy it is to make popcorn on the stove, you may never go back, especially when you realize that one of the biggest benefits is that you get to be in charge of the flavoring (as opposed to microwave bags that often come heavily seasoned with "buttery topping"—who knows what the heck that is?—or something similar).

**3 tablespoons vegetable oil**

**⅓ cup (60 g) popcorn kernels**

**1 tablespoon olive oil**

**1 teaspoon dried oregano**

**1 teaspoon dried rosemary**

**1 teaspoon dried thyme**

**½ teaspoon salt**

1. In a medium saucepan with a tight-fitting lid, melt the oil over medium-high heat.

2. Drop 2 popcorn kernels in the pan and cover. When the kernels pop, the oil is hot enough.

3. Add the remainder of the kernels and promptly cover the pan again. Shake the pan every few seconds to keep the kernels heating evenly and prevent burning.

4. Once the popping slows to less than a few pops per second, take the pan off the heat. Pour the popcorn into a large bowl and drizzle with olive oil, oregano, rosemary, thyme, and salt. Toss well and enjoy.

Per serving: 251 calories, 27.5 g fat (17.5 g saturated fat), 4 g carbs, 582 mg sodium, 1 g fiber, 0 g protein

# RESOURCE GUIDE

There are many books, websites, apps, and more dedicated to helping people banish belly problems. Many of them are awesome and can help you get to the bottom of your issues, figure out what to eat, and more. Others are, well, a load of crap.

I've compiled a list to help you get to some of the good stuff as easily as possible. Of course, there are other great resources out there, but this is a selection of some of my favorites that I think might be valuable to you. Here is the official *A Teen's Guide to Gut Health* Resource Guide, organized by topic; check it out when you're craving more information and ideas.

## GUT HEALTH

### APP

#### MyGiHealth

This cool (and free!) app, developed by experts in the field of digestive diseases and nutrition, uses research-based questionnaires to monitor symptoms and create a GI-focused health history that you can bring to your doctor. Why not skip this step and just go straight to your MD? Well, it can be pretty nerve-racking to tell a near stranger about all of your belly woes. It may, in fact, be easier to talk to your smartphone; according to a study published in the *American Journal of Gastroenterology*, the history compiled by MyGiHealth was more complete and useful than that written by a doctor. Of course, bringing this information to your doctor is the next crucial step. But kicking off the process by tracking your symptoms with MyGiHealth is a smart start.

## BOOKS

*Making Sense of IBS: A Physician Answers Your Questions About Irritable Bowel Syndrome* by Brian E. Lacy (Johns Hopkins University Press, 2013) Written by a doctor and associate professor of medicine at Dartmouth Medical School who specializes in functional gut disorders, this book is a detailed yet readable text about all things IBS. Imagine you spend a long weekend with your gastroenterologist so she can explain the finer points of this disease rather than the fifteen minutes you have in reality. If your GI doc mentions something that you don't understand (LFTs? TCAs?), quick!—make a note (even text it to yourself) and find a thorough explanation in Lacy's book when you get home.

## WEBSITES

International Foundation for Functional Gastrointestinal Disorders
**aboutibs.org**
This nonprofit organization is "dedicated to informing, assisting, and supporting people affected by gastrointestinal disorders." Its website is packed with information about irritable bowel syndrome, from getting diagnosed to

symptoms not to ignore and what to do when your IBS gets in the way of sleep. A must-visit if you have or think you have IBS.

Crohn's & Colitis Foundation of America
**ccfa.org**
This nonprofit is dedicated to finding a cure for Crohn's disease and ulcerative colitis and to improving the quality of life for those diagnosed with the diseases. In addition to information about how to manage IBD, you'll find details about medications you might go on, up-to-the-minute research, and locating a doctor. Another great find on the site: information about fund-raising events like walks, indoor cycling, and half marathon training. Participating (whether as an athlete or a volunteer) can help you feel empowered by taking steps against your disease rather than allowing it to let you feel like a victim.

Just Like Me! Teens with IBD
**justlikemeibd.org**
Managed by the Crohn's & Colitis Foundation of America, this site is written specifically for teenagers who have been diagnosed with inflammatory bowel diseases. My favorite part of this site is the Young Adults Discussion

Forum, a message board where you can post questions and concerns—and offer your support—to other young people with IBD.

## CCFA Campus Connection

**ccfa.org/campus-connection**

Run by the Crohn's & Colitis Foundation of America, this site is devoted to college students and gives pointers on how to prepare for university life, lets you know what you need to think about health care–wise, and even has a scholarship you can apply for (if you've been diagnosed with Crohn's or colitis, that is). There's also a directory to help you connect with other students with IBD at your school.

# LOW-FODMAP DIET AND RECIPES

**BLOG**

## Low FODMAP Diet for Irritable Bowel Syndrome

**fodmapmonash.blogspot.com**

This blog, brought to you by the research team at Monash University that created the low-FODMAP plan, answers questions people have about following the diet, provides recipes, offers information on newly tested foods, and more.

**APP**

## The Monash University Low FODMAP Diet

Possibly the most valuable tool in your low-FODMAP journey and available for iPhone and Android, this app puts a comprehensive food database in your pocket. Look up any of the hundreds—if not thousands—of foods that have been tested by Monash, and the app will tell you if it's a green light (approved), amber (usually OK in very small amounts), or red (avoid). It also features a manual to help guide you through the low-FODMAP diet.

**BOOKS**

*The Complete Low-FODMAP Diet: A Revolutionary Plan for Managing IBS and Other Digestive Disorders* by Sue Shepherd and Peter Gibson (The Experiment Publishing, 2013) Written by the researchers who first developed the low-FODMAP plan, this book is a straightforward guide to the diet along with more than eighty recipes. A no-nonsense read to recommend to your parent or any other adult who wants to understand why you're suddenly being such a picky eater.

**WEBSITE/BLOG**

### The Well Balanced FODMAPer
**blog.katescarlata.com**
Boston-based registered dietitian nutritionist Kate Scarlata went straight to the source—Melbourne, Australia—to learn about the low-FODMAP plan from the very people who pioneered it. She has since helped popularize the low-FODMAP plan in the United States. Her website and blog are full of easy-to-digest (pun intended) information, and the resources she provides (readable lists of high- and low-FODMAP foods and a directory of low-FODMAP-focused registered dietitian nutritionists in the United States and Canada) can make every low-FODMAPer's life easier.

### IBS-Free at Last!
**ibsfree.net**
Maine-based Patsy Catsos has published three books on the low-FODMAP diet and cooking low-FODMAP recipes, based on her ten years of experience learning about and helping people follow the plan (not to mention a trip to the Monash University mothership). Patsy's a wealth of information herself,

and like Kate Scarlata (see previous entry) she also has a directory of FODMAP-literate registered dietitian nutritionists so you can find someone to work with in your area.

# GENERAL NUTRITION/ HEALTH/WELLNESS

**WEBSITES**

### Academy of Nutrition and Dietetics
**eatright.org**
This is the official website of the professional organization that represents the registered dietitian nutritionist profession in the United States. You'll find articles on hot topics in nutrition, how to eat for various health conditions, cooking tips, and more. Use the Find an Expert feature to locate a registered dietitian nutritionist in your area (be sure to ask if he is comfortable with the low-FODMAP plan—or any other diet you're interested in experimenting with).

### MyPlate
**choosemyplate.gov**
Produced by the US Department of Agriculture (USDA), this site provides practical and useful tools for helping you implement MyPlate, the teaching tool

## SILVER LININGS

"I've made friends with girls in my situation."

"My IBS is part of who I am. It's helped me to understand and empathize with other people who may be suffering in their own way. I don't judge people and I try to be the best person I can every day."

"I learned that I have an amazing support network. Since I was diagnosed [with celiac] when I was only four years old, I couldn't make decisions for myself. My mom made it her mission to make me healthy. And it worked!"

"My stress manifested in such a physical way that I was forced to face the things that stress me."

"It gave me good material for a college essay!"

"It's made me a stronger person."

"I have learned a lot about cooking and how strong I am. I now know that I can handle a lot more than I thought I could."

used to help you build a healthier, more balanced meal (see page 118). You'll also find a BMI calculator, a SuperTracker to help you record and analyze your diet, useful articles, and more.

#### MedLine Plus
**medlineplus.gov**
The National Institutes of Health's website for consumers features reliable information about diseases, conditions, and wellness and is produced by the National Library of Medicine.

#### TeensHealth
**kidshealth.org/en/teens**
The teen section of this youth-focused web project from the Nemours Foundation, a nonprofit devoted to children's health, provides young people with honest and accurate information so they can make educated decisions.

# HAVING PERSPECTIVE

"There are people in this world with much worse problems than us!"

"You aren't alone."

"Everyone is dealing with something."

"It gets better."

"If you've gotta go, you gotta go."

Topics include food and fitness, diseases and conditions, sexual health, and mental health.

## The Wellie Project

**thewellieproject.com**

Run by registered dietitian nutritionist and wellness coach Nancy Sidnam, this website's mission is all about "empowering girls to take charge of their health and commit to a life of wellness." The positive self-talk and empowerment woven throughout are exactly what you need when your body hasn't exactly been a good friend to you—but you know you need to show it some love in order to heal. As the website says: "We only get one body, and it needs to last us a lifetime . . . you want to live your best life possible."

## Foodie on Campus

**foodieoncampus.com**

This site bills itself as "the college student's guide to life as a foodie, served with a scoop of nutrition, fitness, and health on the side." It's an excellent resource for college students who are putting some thought into the food they're eating—special diet or not. Foodie on Campus was created and is run by registered dietitian nutritionist Faye Berger Mitchell, who oversees a team of student interns who create content and more. The site is relatable and fun, yet authoritative. Posts are always vetted for accuracy, so you can have complete confidence that you won't be reading about why you should jump on board with the latest "it" diet— thank goodness.

## National Eating Disorders Association

**nationaleatingdisorders.org**

NEDA's mission is to "support individuals and families affected by eating disorders, and serve as a catalyst for prevention, cures, and access to quality care." As you know, there are some links between gut disorders and eating disorders, and undertaking a restrictive diet like the low-FODMAP plan may set the stage for glamorizing limits around food. There's nothing good about eating disorders (of course)—if you think you may be exhibiting disordered eating behavior, this website is a great place to visit to find out what's normal and what's not; it can also help you find help and support.

## National Suicide Prevention Lifeline

**suicidepreventionlifeline.org**

Suicidal thoughts need to be taken seriously. If you're having them, or know someone who is, get help immediately. You can call this organization's 24/7 helpline at 800-273-8255. The website will tell you more about what to expect when you dial the number; it also features valuable information on what to do if someone you care about is in a crisis or exhibiting warning signs.

# LOW-FODMAP FOOD COMPANIES

## MISCELLANEOUS

### FODY Food Co.

**fodyfoods.com**

This US-based company features low-FODMAP foods that have been tested and certified by Monash University in Australia. Products include garlic-infused and onion-infused olive oils, tomato sauce, barbecue sauce, and salsa—delicious flavors that can be near-impossible to come by when you're on a low-FODMAP plan. The company also sells Nicer Foods–branded snack bars. All items are available for ordering online only; the brand currently ships only within the US but is in the process of expanding deliveries to the UK, Canada, and more.

### FODMAPPED for You

**fodmapped.com**

First, the good news: This line of pasta sauces, soups, stocks, and simmer sauces (like green curry and butter chicken—yum!) was created by Sue Shepherd, PhD, an expert on the low-FODMAP plan. So you can rest assured that these flavorful foods are free of onions, garlic, and any other common high-FODMAP ingredients. And now the bad: It's available only in Australia at the time this book was published. We've heard rumors, however, that they might be saying "g'day" to stores on our side of the globe before you know it. Check their website and Facebook page for updates on US distribution.

Rao's Specialty Foods
**raos.com/sensitive-sauce-case**
Yum, yum, and yum. Rao's tomato-based sauces are known for being some of the best around, and their Sensitive sauce formulation, onion-free and garlic-free, is no exception. You can buy it by the case on the Rao's website, which sounds a little crazy until you've tried living without marinara sauce (which you'll have to do if you can't tolerate onions or garlic, because those ingredients are a given in most any jarred sauce).

At around $8 per jar it's not cheap, but it can be a real—and *delizioso*—lifesaver.

# SELECTED BIBLIOGRAPHY

American College of Gastroenterology. "Irritable Bowel Syndrome." Date accessed: September 13, 2016. patients.gi.org/topics/irritable-bowel-syndrome/#

Biesiekierski, Jessica, Simone Peters, Evan Newnham, Ourania Rosella, Jane Muir, and Peter Gibson. "No Effects of Gluten in Patients with Self-Reported Non-Celiac Gluten Sensitivity After Dietary Reduction of Fermentable, Poorly Absorbed, Short-Chain Carbohydrates." *Gastroenterology* 145, no. 2 (August 2013): 320–28.

Catsos, Patsy. *IBS: Free At Last! Change Your Carbs, Change Your Life with the FODMAP Elimination Diet.* 2nd ed. Portland, ME: Pond Cove Press. 2012.

Celiac Disease Foundation. "Screening and Diagnosis." Date accessed: September 4, 2016. celiac.org/celiac-disease/understanding-celiac-disease-2/diagnosing-celiac-disease

Crohn's & Colitis Foundation of America. "Crohn's Disease & Ulcerative Colitis: A Guide For Parents." Date accessed: August 29, 2016. ccfa.org/resources/guide-for-parents.html

Deloose, E., P. Janssen, I. Depoortere, and J. Tack. "The Migrating Motor Complex: Control Mechanisms and Its Role In Health and Disease. *Nature Reviews: Gastroenterology & Hepatology* 9, no. 5 (2012): 271–85.

DiMarino, Michael D. "Overview of the Esophagus." *Merck Manual: Consumer Version.* Date accessed: August 30, 3016. merckmanuals.com/home/digestive-disorders/esophageal-and-swallowing-disorders/overview-of-the-esophagus.

Dukowicz, Andrew C., Brian E. Lacy, and Gary M. Levine. "Small Intestinal Bacterial Overgrowth: A Comprehensive Review." *Gastroenterology & Hepatology* 3, no. 2 (2007): 112–22.

Fedewa, A., and S. S. C. Rao. "Dietary Fructose Intolerance, Fructan Intolerance and FODMAPs." *Current Gastroenterology Reports* 16, no. 1 (2014): 370.

Frank, L., L. Kleinman, A. Rentz, G. Ciesla, J. J. Kim, and C. Zacker. "Health-Related Quality of Life Associated with Irritable Bowel Syndrome: Comparison with Other Chronic Diseases." *Clinical Therapeutics* 24, no. 4 (April 2002).

Halmos, Emma, Claus Christophersen, Anthony Bird, Susan Shepherd, Peter Gibson, and Jane Muir. "Diets That Differ in Their FODMAP Content Alter the Colonic Luminal Microenvironment." *Gut* 64, no. 1 (2015): 93–100.

Hulisz, Darrell. "The Burden of Illness of Irritable Bowel Syndrome: Current Challenges and Hope for the Future." *Journal of Managed Care Pharmacy* 10, no. 4 (2004): 299–309.

Hungin, A. P. S., L. Chang, G. R. Locke, E. H. Dennis, and V. Barghout. "Irritable Bowel Syndrome in the United States: Prevalence, Symptom Patterns, and Impact." *Alimentary Pharmacology & Therapeutics* 2, no. 11 (2005): 1365–75.

Hyams, J. S., G. Burke, P. M. Davis, B. Rzepski, and P. A. Andrulonis. "Abdominal Pain and Irritable Bowel Syndrome in Adolescents: A Community Based Study." *Journal of Pediatrics* 129, no. 2 (1996): 220-26.

Lacy, Brian E. *Making Sense of IBS: A Physician Answers Your Questions About Irritable Bowel Syndrome.* 2nd ed. Baltimore: Johns Hopkins University Press, 2013. Pages 54–55; 264–65.

Maggard, Louise, Dorit V. Ankerson, and Pia Munkholm. "Follow-Up of Patients with Functional Bowel Symptoms Treated with a Low FODMAP Diet." *World Journal of Gastroenterology* 22, no. 15 (2016): 4009–19.

Mahan, Kathleen L., and Janice L. Raymond. *Krause's Food & The Nutrition Care Process.* 14th ed. St. Louis, MO: Elsevier, 2017. Pages 7; 13–15

Miskovitz, Paul, and Marian Betancourt. *The Doctor's Guide to Gastrointestinal Health: Preventing and Treating Acid Reflux, Ulcers, Irritable Bowel Syndrome, Diverticulitis, Celiac Disease, Colon Cancer, Pancreatitis, Cirrhosis, Hernias, and More.* Hoboken, NJ: John Wiley & Sons, 2005. Pages 80–81.

National Institute of Diabetes and Digestive and Kidney Disorders. "Your Digestive System and How It Works." Date accessed: August 29, 2016. niddk.nih.gov/health-information/health-topics/Anatomy/your-digestive-system/Pages/anatomy.aspx

Pimentel, M., E. J. Chow, and H. C. Lin. "Normalization of Lactulose Breath Testing Correlates with Symptom Improvement in Irritable Bowel Syndrome: A Double-Blind, Randomized, Placebo-Controlled Study." *American Journal of Gastroenterology* 98, no. 2 (2003): 412–19.

Rasquin, Andre, Carlo Di Lorenzo, David Forbes, Ernesto Guiraldes, Jeffrey S. Hyams, Annamaria Staiano, and Lynn S. Walker. "Childhood Functional Gastrointestinal Disorders: Child/Adolescent." *Gastroenterology* 130, no. 5 (2006): 1527–37.

Scarlata, Kate. *Low FODMAP 28-Day Plan: A Healthy Cookbook with Gut Friendly Recipes for IBS Relief.* Berkeley, CA: Rockridge Press, 2014.

Shepherd, Sue, and Peter Gibson. *The Complete Low-FODMAP Diet. A Revolutionary Plan for Managing IBS and Other Digestive Disorders.* New York: The Experiment, 2013. Page 35.

Shepherd, Susan, and Peter Gibson. "Fructose Malabsorption and Symptoms of Irritable Bowel Syndrome: Guidelines for Effective Dietary Management." *Journal of the Academy of Nutrition and Dietetics* 106, no. 10 (2006): 1631–39.

Tamborlane, William, and Janet Weiswasser. *The Yale Guide to Children's Nutrition.* New Haven, CT: Yale University Press, 1997. Pages 10–11.

The Rome Foundation. "What's New for Rome IV." Date accessed: September 14, 2016. theromefoundation.org/rome-iv/whats-new-for-rome-iv

Triantafyllou, Konstantinos, Christopher Chang, and Mark Pimentel. "Methanogens, Methane, and Gastrointestinal Motility." *Journal of Neurogastroenterology and Motility* 20, no. 1 (2014): 31–40.

Whitney, Ellie, and Sharon Rady Rolfes. *Understanding Nutrition.* 11th ed. Belmont, CA: Thomson Higher Education, 2007. Pages 87, 108–109.

# ACKNOWLEDGMENTS

This book would not exist without the hard work and support of many people.

Thank you to Sue Shepherd, PhD, and Peter Gibson, MD, for developing the low-FODMAP plan—you have helped so many people, and I'm so honored to help your work reach teens. Much appreciation as well goes to the gastroenterology department at Monash University for continuing this fascinating research and for sharing its knowledge with the public.

To the registered dietitian nutritionists who are responsible for popularizing the low-FODMAP diet in the United States: Kate Scarlata, RDN, and Patsy Catsos, MS, RD, LD. Your mission to teach other RDNs about this revolutionary plan means that you have improved the lives of more people than you can ever imagine. I've learned so much from your trainings, lectures, books, and blog posts. Thank you for your wisdom and generosity.

To the RMW Nutrition interns who have helped me at various stages of writing this book—Hillary Pasternak, Denise Ulloa, and Leah Negrin. I'm also appreciative of Jenna Pasternak and Hannah Plotka for not laughing at me when I asked, "Do teenagers really say _____?" and for babysitting so I could stay (sort of) on my deadlines, respectively.

I am so thankful to my friend and colleague Cynthia Sass, MPH, MA, RD, CSSD, who is always there when I need her with professional guidance or a laugh. I'm also lucky to have supportive friends and colleagues like Teresa Dumain, Kerri-Ann Jennings, Melissa Gallagher, Naava Katz, Anne Mauney, Leah Mermelstein, Terra Schmookler Fuhr, and Stephanie Weiss, all of the Tufts Nutrition Superheroes, and everyone in the extended Meltzer and Warren families cheering me along the way (and understanding when it takes me months to return a phone call—sorry!).

Thank you to the amazing team at The Experiment who saw the need for a book like this and helped me every step along the way—Jennifer Hergenroeder, Matthew Lore, Batya Rosenblum, Jeanne Tao, Sarah Smith, Vivienne Woodward, and especially Allie Bochicchio for believing in the idea, Jennifer Boudinot for carefully polishing my words and making sure my teen culture references are on point (on fleek?), and Joan Strasbaugh for seeing it through to publication. Thanks also to Becky Terhune for designing a book that makes stomach problems feel fun and exciting to read about. Thank you as well to my fantastic agent, Danielle Chiotti, for helping me transform my rambling ideas into books, and for turning my childhood dream of becoming an author into a reality.

I blame everything I am on my parents, Janet and Michael. Thank you to them for guiding, backing, and loving me. My brother, Daniel, is my in-house photographer and always a text away, and for that I am thankful.

And finally, thank you to my chosen family: Scott, who has endured many late nights and working weekends while I bond with my MacBook. Words cannot adequately express my appreciation of you. Liliana, thank you for "writing" Chapter 5 for me (in crayon) and for drawing pictures of me giving kids fruits and vegetables while I typed—for someone who can make it pretty hard to get work done, you help and inspire me every day.

# INDEX

colitis, ulcerative, 33–34

college, low-FODMAP plan in, 101–4

colon, 8–9

condiments, 58, 59, 61, 65, 81

cooking, 91, 94–96, 99, 134

Crohn's disease, 32–33

Culturelle (*Lactobacillus GG*), 130

# D

dairy/dairy alternatives, 56, 59, 60–61, 63

dating, 103

depression, 125

diagnostic tests, 19–26

diet options

    autoimmune Paleo diet, 48–49

    blood-type diet, 51

    GAPS protocol, 50

    gluten-free diet, 46–48

    grain-free diet, 48

    low-residue/low-fiber diet, 50–51

    Paleo diet, 48

    specific carbohydrate diet, 49–50

    *See also* low-FODMAP plan

digestion, 3–10

    eating, 4–5

    GI tract overview, 3–4

    intestines, 7–9

    pooping, 7

    stomach, 5–7

    supporting players, 9–10

diners, 76

dining halls/cafeterias, 76–82, 98–101

dinner, 67, 79

disaccharides, 44

disordered eating, 124, 126–27

doctors, 11–13, 18–19, 131

    *See also* tests, diagnostic

dorm room food, 77

double boilers, 185

duodenum, 7

dysbiosis, 129

# E

eating, in digestion, 4–5

eating disorders, 124, 126–27

eating out, 70–82

    children's menus, 72

    dining halls/cafeterias, 76–82, 98–101

    restaurant types, 72–76

    survival guide, 70–71

elimination phase, 83–84

emergencies, medical, 11–12

endoscopy, upper, 22

enema, 23

enterography, magnetic resonance, 26

enteroscopy, balloon-assisted, 22

erythritol, 63

esophagus, 5

events, surviving big, 132

exams, school, 142

exercise, 139

# F

fast food restaurants, 74

fats, 58, 109, 116–18

fecal microbiota transplant (FMT), 135

fermentable, as term, 43

fermented foods, 132–36

fiber, 121, 130

flavor, boosting, 69–70

flexible sigmoidoscopy, 24–25

FMT (fecal microbiota transplant), 135

FODMAP, as term, 43–45

    *See also* low-FODMAP plan

food-service directors, 99–101, 102–4

friends, 103

fructans, 62

fructo-oligosaccharides (FOS), 44

fructose, 44–45

fructose intolerance breath test, 21

fructose malabsorption/intolerance, 36–37

fruit, 56, 59, 60, 64–65, 69, 113–14, 121

functional gut disorders, 28

    *See also* irritable bowel syndrome

## G

galacto-oligosaccharides, 44

GAPS (gut and psychology syndrome) protocol, 50

garlic, 62, 80

gastric emptying scan (GES), 25

gastroenterologists, 18–19

gastrointestinal motility, 31

gastrointestinal tract overview, 3–4

genetics, 30

GI docs, 18–19

GI tract overview, 3–4

gluten-free diet, 46–48, 60

Go foods, 53, 55–58, 61–65

Go Low. *See* low-FODMAP plan

Go Low phase 1, 83–84

Go Low phase 2, 85–86, 88–91

grain-free diet, 49

grains and cereals, 62–63, 112–13, 123

grazing, 10

Greek restaurants, 75–76

grocery shopping, 61–65, 91–92, 93

gut and psychology syndrome (GAPS) protocol, 50

gut-brain connection, 137–44

gut-brain miscommunication, 30

gut-directed biofeedback, 144

gut-directed hypnotherapy, 143–44

gut-food connection, 39–41

## H

health insurance, 27

high school, low-FODMAP plan in, 97–101

hypnotherapy, gut-directed, 143–44

## I

IBS (irritable bowel syndrome), 27–32

Indian restaurants, 75

inflammatory bowel disease (IBD), 32–33

    *See also* Crohn's disease; ulcerative colitis

In-N-Out Burger, 74

insurance, health, 27

intestines, 7–9, 31

irritable bowel syndrome (IBS), 27–32

Italian restaurants, 72

## J

Japanese restaurants, 72–73

Jimmy John's restaurants, 74

journals, food/symptom, 84, 86–87

nonceliac gluten sensitivity (NCGS), 46–47

nutrition

    antioxidants, 110–11

    calories, 109, 111–12

    defined, 105

    facts versus fiction, 106–8

    macronutrients, 109, 111–19

    micronutrients, 109–10

    MyPlate, 118–20

nutritionists, registered dietitian, 2, 89, 107, 108, 131

nuts and seeds, 58, 59, 61, 64, 118, 123, 124

## O

oils, 58, 115, 118, 121–22

oligosaccharides, 43–44

onions, 62, 70–71, 80

opioid abuse, 125

## P

packaged-food ingredients, 61

Paleo diet, 48

Panera Bread, 74

parents, talking with, 15–18

PCPs (primary care providers), 18

perfectionism, 122

peristalsis, 5, 7, 8

planning ahead, 96–97

polyols, 4

pooping, 7

poop transplants, 135

portion size, 53, 54, 90–91

power packs, 97

prebiotics, 129, 130–36

primary care providers (PCPs), 18

probiotics, 129, 130–36

protein

    in low-FODMAP plan, 57, 59, 60, 61, 63–64, 68, 114–16

    as macronutrient, 109, 114–16

    for vegetarians/vegans, 122–24

protein powder, 116

PubMed, 107–8

## R

rectum, 9

referral to gastroenterologist, 18

registered dietitian nutritionists, 2, 89, 107, 108, 131

reintroduction phase, 85–86, 88–91

research, 107–8

restaurants, 70–76

## S

salad bars, 81–82

salad dressings, 80, 81

salads, cold, 68

salivary amylase, 4

salivation, 4

sandwiches, 68

saturated fats, 117–18

sauces, 80

sauerkraut, 133–34

SCD (specific carbohydrate diet), 49–50

school survival tips, 13

seeds and nuts, 58, 59, 61, 64, 118, 123, 124

seitan, 124

shopping, grocery, 61–65, 91–92

Slow foods, 53, 59

small intestinal bacterial overgrowth (SIBO), 37–38

small intestinal bacterial overgrowth (SIBO) breath test, 21–22

small intestine, 7–8

snacks, 64, 67, 96, 101, 121

social life, 103

soups, 80

sources, evaluating, 106

sourdough bread, 136

soy, 123

specific carbohydrate diet (SCD), 49–50

spiralizers, 168

Starbucks, 74

steak houses, 76

stomach, 5–7

stool analysis, 20

stool transplantation, 135

stress, 30, 138, 143

sugar alcohols, 4

sugars, simple, 113

suicide, 125–26

sweeteners, 63, 114

symptoms

    about, 11–12

    talking about, 16

    tracking, 13–15

## T

talking to others, 14, 15–18, 127

talk therapy, 142

teachers, 102

tempeh, 123, 134

tests, diagnostic, 19–26

Thai restaurants, 73, 75

toasted bread, 69

trans fats, 117

## U

ulcerative colitis, 33–34

upper endoscopy, 22

upper GI and small bowel series, 25–26

## V

vegetables, 55–56, 59, 60, 64–65, 69, 113–14, 118

vegetarians and vegans, 122–23

villi, 7–8

visceral hypersensitivity, 31

VSL#3, 131

## W

Waffle House, 74

weight, healthy, 110

Wendy's restaurants, 74

## X

x-rays, 25

## Y

yoga, 141

yogurt, 133

# RECIPE INDEX

# NOTES

# NOTES

# ABOUT THE AUTHOR

RACHEL MELTZER WARREN, MS, RDN, is a nutrition writer, educator, and counselor who makes healthy eating delicious, easy, fun, and fashionable. The author of *The Smart Girl's Guide to Going Vegetarian* book and blog, she has a BA in magazine journalism from the University of Maryland, College Park, and has written for *Women's Health*, *Shape*, *Vegetarian Times*, *Good Housekeeping*, and others. She's also a registered dietitian nutritionist (RDN) with an MS in nutrition communication from the Friedman School of Nutrition Science and Policy at Tufts University. Rachel lives in Jersey City, New Jersey, where she counsels others in eating well and consults for educational programs such as the Harlem Children's Zone, developing and teaching classes on nutrition and wellness. You can find her online at www.rmwnutrition.com or twitter.com/RMWnutrition.